Biomedicalization and the
Practice of Culture

STUDIES IN SOCIAL MEDICINE

Allan M. Brandt, Larry R. Churchill, and Jonathan Oberlander, editors

This series publishes books at the intersection of medicine, health, and society that further our understanding of how medicine and society shape one another historically, politically, and ethically. The series is grounded in the convictions that medicine is a social science, that medicine is humanistic and cultural as well as biological, and that it should be studied as a social, political, ethical, and economic force.

Biomedicalization and the Practice of Culture

Globalization and Type 2 Diabetes in the United States and Japan

Mari Armstrong-Hough

University of North Carolina Press CHAPEL HILL

This book was published with the assistance of the Lilian R. Furst Fund of the University of North Carolina Press.

The University of North Carolina Press has been a member of the
Green Press Initiative since 2003.

Library of Congress Cataloging-in-Publication Data
Names: Armstrong-Hough, Mari, author.
Title: Biomedicalization and the practice of culture : globalization and type 2 diabetes in the
    United States and Japan / Mari Armstrong-Hough.
Other titles: Studies in social medicine.
Description: Chapel Hill : University of North Carolina Press, [2018] | Series: Studies in social
    medicine | Includes bibliographical references and index.
Identifiers: LCCN 2018019133| ISBN 9781469646671 (cloth : alk. paper) | ISBN 9781469646688
    (pbk : alk. paper) | ISBN 9781469646695 (ebook)
Subjects: LCSH: Non-insulin-dependent diabetes—United States. | Non-insulin-dependent
    diabetes—Japan. | Non-insulin-dependent Diabetes—Treatment—United States. |
    Non-insulin-dependent Diabetes—Treatment—Japan. | Non-insulin-dependent
    diabetes—Social Aspects—United States. | Non-insulin-dependent diabetes—
    Social Aspects—Japan.
Classification: LCC RC662.18 .A78 2018 | DDC 362.1964/624—dc23 LC record available at
    https://lccn.loc.gov/2018019133

Cover illustrations: *Vial and Syringe* © iStock.com/Sezeryadigar; *Pille Background*
© iStock.com/Sohl.

For my family, here and away

Contents

Acknowledgments

My families in the United States and Japan had to live with me all these years, and in their persevering patience made this project possible: to the entire Armstrong-Hough-Nelson-Edes clan and Remes-Carliner family, thank you. Thank you especially to Drs. Takaaki and Kazue Matsuo, our chosen family and the reason Okayama became home.

Many guides, mentors, and collaborators made this research possible. Thank you especially to Dr. Okamura, Dr. Junichi Nakahara, Dr. Daisaku Dairokuno, Dr. Wasa Fujii, Dr. Ayami Nakatani, Dr. Takahashi, Dr. Megumi Oda, the Suga family, and the Okada family. Thank you to approximately a hundred unnamed physicians, nurse practitioners, and nurses who took time out of their overwhelming schedules to talk with me about their work. I would not have been able to begin, much less finish, without Dr. Linda George, Dr. Lynn Smith-Lovin, Dr. Nan Lin, Dr. Leo Ching, Dr. Anne Allison, Dr. Ed Tiryakian, or Dr. Suzanne Shanahan. Dr. Kazumi Hatasa, Dr. Chie Muramatsu, Dr. Miura, and the rest of the Middlebury Japanese Language School worked their magic two years in a row. Three anonymous reviewers strengthened the first draft of the manuscript with their questions and criticisms. My amazing students and research assistants at Meiji University, especially Yuma Nambu, Manami Hakoda, Shiro Furuya, and Hideaki Tonoike, made the second round of research for this book during three years in Tokyo interesting and productive. Thank you to all members of the Japan Multigenerational Interview Project who critiqued early versions of this project, contributed to interview guides, worked to recruit participants, and assisted with or carried out interviews: Juichi Suzuki, Shin Yonesaka, Anna Maki, Hiroaki Yamada, Hideaki Tonoike, Sarasa Hayashi, Yutaro Takeuchi, Yasuhisa N., Yuto Oshima, Ayuko Takeda, Tomoka Yamada, Daiki Yanai, Tomoya Abe, Taiga Aoki, Than Htay Aung, Yamato Fujisawa, Satoru Goshi, Yukiko Homma, Mitsuki Imamura, Takayuki Ishikawa, Yuki Ishiyama, Kensuke Matsumoto, Michiko Mitsuta, Ayano Nakagawa, Yuma Nambu, Natsuki Inoue, Jun Ono, Ryu Ru, Junichi Sakata, Yuki Tamatsuka, Toru Taniguchi, Kazuaki Tanikawa, and Takumi Wakimura.

This research would not have been possible without significant financial support from the Asian Pacific Studies Institute at Duke University, the

Foreign Language and Area Studies (FLAS) Fellowship, and the faculty research fund of the School of Political Science and Economics at Meiji University in Tokyo.

I owe a further debt of gratitude to many friends and colleagues who shared their insights over several years: Mariko Suga, Yuka Nagata, Jill Powers, Jessica Rubenstein, Emily Mills, Shiro Furuya, Teresa Umeki, Yasuaki Umeki, Kieran Rance, Peyton Bowman, Riley Smith, Colette Wiffen, Helen Matsubara, Naomi Sharlin, Fitzalan Crowe, Kim Rogers, Mitch Fraas, Abhijit Mehta, Karen Rembold, Sarah Heilbronner, Ben Hayden, Irene Liu, Matt and Jenny Crowley, Erika Alpert, Yoshinori Hananoi, Toshie Okada, Yuriko Okada, and the wombats (Basuberi-san, Zaara-san, Sebura-san, and Oh-san).

I wish I could thank my dog, Rutherford, but I think his long adolescence probably delayed this book by at least a year. He is a good boy anyway.

Finally, thank you to Jacob Remes, who moved to the *inaka*, braved a language he never intended to learn, and ended up falling in love with Okayama (and marrying me). I never would have finished this project without him.

Biomedicalization and the Practice of Culture

Introduction
Two Countries, One Disease

It was the middle of winter, and I was sitting in a narrow classroom with an institutional linoleum floor, fluorescent lights, and windows overlooking a parking lot. Fifteen or so students, mostly men over the age of 40, sat uncomfortably at long tables facing a whiteboard, on which a nurse had drawn several figures illustrating insulin receptors. Having finished her explanation, she was erasing the figures.

"Next, let's talk about food," she said in crisp, authoritative Japanese. "Please turn to page 38 in your books."

We obediently flipped through the pages of our hospital-issued textbooks until we came to a page with pictures of several different meals, accompanied by nutritional information.

"Well, what are good foods?"

A gaunt man in a work jumpsuit raised his hand. "Vegetables," he said.

"Rice!" said a woman in the back.

"Japanese foods," said another.

"*Konnyaku.*"

The nurse nodded in approval and launched into a practical explanation of healthy meal planning for the management of type 2 diabetes. She pointed to the photographed examples of appropriately balanced and portioned breakfasts, lunches, and dinners. Every meal pictured included a small bowl of rice.

A little while later, the nurse prompted us for "danger" foods.

"What should we be careful of?" she asked.

"Fried foods."

"*Western* foods."

"Eating out."

"Beer and sake, things like that."

An elderly man to my right turned and looked at me forlornly. Even though I was crammed uncomfortably behind a table like the other students, I wore my white lab coat and a hospital identification badge.

"But it's okay to drink a little sake, right?" he asked hopefully.

* * *

RATES OF TYPE 2 DIABETES rose rapidly in Japan during the last years of the twentieth century. By the early 2000s, nearly one in five Japanese had impaired glucose tolerance, a precursor to diabetes (MHLW 2007). In a nationally representative sample, more than 17 percent of men and nearly 10 percent of women over the age of thirty met standard diagnostic thresholds for type 2 diabetes in Japan (MHLW 2012). Prevalence increases with age: more than 22 percent of men over sixty and more than 16 percent of women over seventy had hemoglobin A1c (HbA1c) levels over Japan's 6.1 percent threshold for diagnosing diabetes (MHLW 2010: 6). As Japan has grayed, its diabetes epidemic has grown.

Most Americans are surprised to hear that type 2 diabetes is epidemic in Japan, a nation popularly associated with healthy food and small body mass. To be sure, age-adjusted rates of diabetes are higher in the United States than in Japan. More than a quarter of Americans over sixty-five have diabetes (CDC 2011). But the U.S. population is younger than that of Japan, and rates for younger Americans and Japanese are similar, particularly among males. Diabetes affects just 9 percent of all Americans over the age of eighteen (CDC 2012), a smaller proportion of the total adult population than are affected in Japan. By the 2000s, both countries faced serious and rapidly expanding epidemics.

Japan experienced many of the same social and economic changes over the last century that drove rising rates of diabetes in the United States: increased availability of cheap processed foods, changing portion sizes, sedentary work and recreation patterns, reliance on motorized transportation, tobacco use, economic inequality, and longer life spans. Moreover, as almost any type 2 diabetes patient in Japan is eager to point out, Japanese, along with many people of Asian descent, may inherit greater risk for the condition as a result of physiological differences (Chan et al. 2009). When matched by age, body mass index (BMI), waist circumference, and diet, healthy individuals of Asian descent have higher postprandial glucose levels and lower insulin sensitivity (Dickinson et al. 2002). This higher risk for diabetes among people of Asian descent may be related to a tendency to deposit visceral fat and to a genetic predisposition for a pancreatic beta-cell abnormality that influences insulin resistance (Chan et al. 2009). Japan's diabetes patients reflect this pattern, including large numbers of the "metabolically" but not conventionally obese: patients who have a normal BMI by conventional ranges, but increased abdominal adiposity.

As its population aged, Japan's policymakers worried that the diabetes epidemic, along with a host of other so-called lifestyle diseases, could threaten the soundness of the Japanese health care system.[1] Japan enjoys one of the most cost-efficient health care systems in the world, but the specter of widespread chronic disease and an aging population threatens to bankrupt that system.[2] In 2001, the Ministry of Health, Labor, and Welfare (MHLW) introduced Health Japan 21, a bundle of public health promotion programs aimed at primary or secondary prevention of noncommunicable diseases, including type 2 diabetes (Sakurai 2003; Ma et al. 2017). Similar to target-setting public health programs like Healthy People 2000 in the United States, the Health Japan 21 objectives focused on primary prevention of lifestyle diseases. "We should not limit our effort only to early detection through routine medical examination, which is the basis of traditional disease control," wrote a group of the plan's architects (Shibaike et al. 2002).

As part of this initiative, the MHLW rolled out an unprecedented national screening program for diabetes, prediabetes, and its precursor, metabolic syndrome, in April 2008 (Udagawa, Miyoshi & Yoshiike 2008).[3] Because visceral fat is associated with risk for diabetes, the ratio of waist girth to hip girth is a fast and inexpensive primary screening tool. The ministry thus set out to measure the waist of *every Japanese worker* in workplaces and city health centers. City governments struggled to meet an ambitious target: measure the waistlines of at least 65 percent of their eligible residents. Men with waists larger than 33.5 inches and women with waists larger than 33.4 inches were referred to a physician for dietary education and testing. The objective was to identify and manage incipient diabetes before it started by providing medical counsel and intensified monitoring to the most immediately at-risk individuals—those with prediabetes, metabolic syndrome, or other major risk factors. Doing so may not prevent diabetes from eventually developing (primary prevention), but early intervention may slow the disease's progression and prevent complications (secondary prevention). In one stroke, the MHLW applied a pre-illness identity based on risk for diabetes to approximately 14 million Japanese.

The measuring-tape scheme proved cheap, safe, effective, and relatively uncontroversial, though it only reached around 40 percent of those targeted. But American newspaper articles describing the initiative portrayed the national waist-measuring effort as quirky and Japanese rather than as a potentially imitable public health measure.[4] It was inconceivable that such a screening intervention be implemented in the United States, a nation facing an even more serious epidemic, where the average diabetes patient is said to go up to seven years without a diagnosis. Aside from the institutional differences between the two countries, the mass semipublic measurement of waists by public health workers would seriously offend American sensibilities. Lining up American workers in their own workplaces and wrapping a tape measure around their middles seemed not just laughable but intrusive—even a little disgusting.

The sense of *possibility* for public health interventions is very different between the United States and Japan, even for the same disease. These differences, of course, grow in part from institutional differences in the organization of health care delivery. But they also arise from differences in what the general public (and medical community) will tolerate from public health authorities. Different conceptualizations of appropriate and inappropriate uses of the body—and different assumptions about who is responsible for maintaining the body—create very different possibilities for public health interventions. Different cultural tool kits (Swidler 1986) provide different materials for building strategies in response to the same epidemic.

The differences between American and Japanese approaches to diabetes extend well beyond government efforts to measure the girth of the Japanese public. The ways in which physicians describe and treat the disease, and the ways in which patients explain its origins and prevention, reveal empirical differences between experiences and care for diabetes in the two countries. The diabetes education session described at the beginning of this chapter touched on a few of those differences. The recommendation that white rice should be eaten at most meals, for instance, would not make it into an American diabetes education session. Quite the opposite, most American health professionals recommend that their patients minimize white rice consumption—many go so far as to say it should be avoided entirely.

The emphasis on the particular danger of foreign foods may also seem odd in an American context. Most Americans are under the (quite possibly accurate) impression that nothing is unhealthier than American food. But Mediterranean diets, Southeast Asian cuisines, Indian food, and other "foreign" food traditions popular in the United States are not portrayed as particularly dangerous to the health of the American people. Rather, the twin epidemics of obesity and diabetes are perceived to be homegrown—literally—in the cornfields of Middle America. In Japan, however, foreign foods—including dishes associated with Mediterranean diets—are implicated in the rise of diabetes in popular discourse.

Further differences emerge in clinical settings. Outpatients with type 2 diabetes in Japan are seen by physicians much more frequently than their counterparts in the United States. This is in line with broader differences in health care utilization between the two countries: Organisation for Economic

Co-operation and Development (OECD) data show that the average American patient has around four health visits per year, while the average Japanese patient has more than thirteen health visits annually. At minimum, patients with type 2 diabetes in Japan are expected to visit the outpatient clinic once every two months, but most are seen at least once a month. Nearly a quarter of the diabetes patients at the suburban hospital where I did my fieldwork were seen for five-minute check-in visits once every two weeks. In contrast, the American Diabetes Association (ADA) recommends that type 2 diabetes patients be seen by a doctor only once every two months. And most Americans with diabetes — even those with reasonably good insurance — do not go nearly that often (Spann et al. 2006). These differences undoubtedly emerge directly from major differences in the organization and finance of the Japanese and American health systems. But they also contribute to dramatic differences in the experience of diabetes care among patients and in the culture of clinical management among providers.

When it comes to frequency of health visits for diagnosed type 2 diabetes patients, the gold standard in the United States is considered to be the bare minimum in Japan. When physicians at an urban welfare hospital in Japan explained to me that most of their type 2 diabetes visit only once every two months, they seemed almost apologetic. "We're just too busy here," explained one internist I shadowed at the bustling downtown medical center. To him, seeing diabetes patients only once every other month was regrettable, even mildly embarrassing.

Physicians' prescription choices for diabetes patients also vary across the two countries. The majority of prescription pharmaceuticals in Japan are still dispensed by physicians, a system that is widely understood to distort prescription choices in favor of overmedication (Iizuka 2007). However, in the case of type 2 diabetes, Japanese physicians are actually *less* likely to prescribe medication and more likely to favor lifestyle modification than American physicians, especially shortly after diagnosis.

Once in the Japanese exam room, many parts of the consultation would be familiar to those who have spent time in American diabetes clinics: the physician will discuss HbA1c and fasting blood glucose (FBG) values, note the patient's weight, discuss lifestyle factors, and adjust medication. A large part of the short exam will be given over to diabetes education — that is, explaining the disease, its implications, and strategies for self-care. But other aspects of the Japanese exam will seem unusual. In suburban and rural clinics, patients self-report their weight; no nurse will weigh them. Many patients at the diabetes clinic do not have diabetes at all, but rather impaired glucose tolerance (IGT), metabolic syndrome, or some other risk factor for diabetes. Most patients will carry a *techou*, a small notebook in which they have carefully recorded daily food intake. Patients may be admitted to the hospital for the sole purpose of behavior and lifestyle training or modification. Occasionally, a physician will declare a patient cured. Because Japan pursued its own standardization program for HbA1c beginning in the 1990s, the diagnostic reference values for diabetes and prediabetes differed substantially from those used in the United States and Europe until 2013 (Little & Rohlfing 2009; Kashiwagi et al. 2012; Amemiya & Hoshino 2013; Ishibashi 2013); the clinician may thus share two different HbA1c values with different interpretations. And, of course, the recommendations for meal planning will differ significantly.

To manage the same chronic disease, physicians in Japan recommend portion-controlled rice and fish, while American providers prefer to recommend low-carbohydrate diets and warn against white rice. Japanese physicians emphasize frequent contact with a physician, while more and more patients in the United States are served by nurse practitioners (or not at all). Japanese physicians encourage their patients to maintain careful diet records, while American physicians favor a "broad strokes" approach. Physicians in Japan emphasize immediate, major lifestyle modification to manage blood sugar, while American physicians depend more on medication to achieve and sustain glycemic control. Even the diagnostic threshold for type 2 diabetes differs between the two countries: related to the population risk differences discussed earlier, the Japan Diabetes Society opts for a lower threshold, diagnosing the disease earlier in its progression and setting lower HbA1c targets (Neville et al. 2009). All of these differences reflect different philosophies of care, different expectations about how health is maintained and illness kept at bay, and different assumptions about who is responsible for health outcomes.

How do we approach such differences? Both health care systems emphasize evidence-based medicine, operate in technologically advanced societies, and are manned by cosmopolitan professionals who reference international guidelines. Elite Japanese physicians complete research fellowships abroad and publish in international, English-language medical journals. They cite the recommendations of international and American institutions like the ADA and CDC even as they enact clinical practices that differ substantially from those in the United States.

Japan has a long tradition of empirical medical research. Its physicians are embedded in global professional networks that connect them to American counterparts. Yet their ideas about best practices in medicine differ from standard American practice. Further, laypeople in the two countries talk about the origins of the epidemic and illness experiences in profoundly different ways. Japanese patients give one another different advice regarding the prevention of diabetes and imagine health maintenance differently from their American counterparts. These differences relate directly to different patient behavior, different forms of provider-patient relationships, and different approaches to the biomedical treatment of type 2 diabetes.

In the following chapters, I examine how and why clinicians in both Japan and the United States enact empirical biomedical practices that they perceive to be universal — in ways that are decidedly local. Health care providers in both contexts act on the basis of increasingly globalized professional standards. But they also rely on local knowledge, on their own explanatory models for type 2 diabetes, and on local patient populations' explanatory models in their efforts to reach clinical decisions and communicate them to patients. In this way, local knowledge and localized interactions with patients shape the ways in which practicing physicians interpret global standards and best practices. The interaction of globalizing standards of practice, local knowledge, and local explanatory models results in dramatically divergent practices across different social contexts.

I call this the *durability* of distinct medical cultures. In technologically advanced health care systems that rely on evidence-based approaches to producing new medical knowledge, distinct medical cultures persist. Professionals and patients maintain or develop anew meaningfully different practices and illness narratives — even as increasing consensus seems to be pressing health practices toward a single global standard. The following chapters demonstrate how distinctive practices endure in approaches to type 2 diabetes in the United States and Japan, both on the part of patients and on the part of their physicians. Furthermore, they demonstrate the roles that local knowledge, local explanatory models, and local discourses about the origins of the diabetes epidemic play in shaping health practices in each context, making cultures of practice remarkably resilient in the face of technological globalization.

Medicine as a Social Enterprise

The insight that social structure and culture imprint health practices is well established. American sociologists have analyzed the institutional origins of medical prestige (Starr 1982), the social and political processes by which diseases are defined (Conrad & Schneider 1992; Conrad 2005; Conrad & Leiter 2004), and the fundamental social causes of the distribution of disease in our society (Link & Phelan 1995; see also Aneshensel 1992; George 1996; House et al. 1994). Decades of scholarship show that culture plays an important role not only in how doctors' advice is understood but also in the actual content of that advice (Waitzkin 1989; Schouten et al. 2007). Others have found that socioeconomic and cultural gaps between doctors and patients in the United States result in different levels of health care utilization between social groups (Andersen 1995), in differences in prescription rates of analgesics (Tamayo-Sarver et al. 2003), in misunderstanding and hostility between patients and providers (Abrums 2000), and occasionally in tragic failures of communication (Fadiman 1997). Medical anthropologists have explored the underpinnings and implications of variation in illness narratives across communities (Hunt et al. 1998, 2002).

This body of work has established that culture, broadly defined, plays an important role in medical practice. However, it offers little leverage for explaining the relationship between medical systems and cultures outside Europe and North America. While it demonstrates that culture is a resource in biomedical encounters, without the perspective provided by explicitly comparative work we lack a sense of its contours. We often fail to fully theorize the pathways from cultural context to behavior. Moreover, discussions of culture in biomedical literature have historically treated culture as an attribute of the patient, rather than of the encounter with the patient.

The relative lack of comparative studies of the practice of evidence-based biomedicine in non-U.S. or European settings and countries not only prevents us from understanding other medical systems, it prevents us from fully understanding even the systems we do study. This book seeks to fill that gap by engaging in comparative analysis of narratives, experiences, and practices surrounding a single disease—type 2 diabetes—in two technologically advanced, high-resource settings with high rates of the same chronic disease—the United States and Japan.

Social institutions also profoundly shape medicine. Paul Starr's classic work traced the institutional origins of American medicine, exposing the ways in which professionalization shaped American medicine (Starr 1982). Institutional arrangements define the opportunity structure in which medicalization theorists identify the politics of disease definition (Conrad & Schneider 1992; Brown 1995; Light 2000a). And a comparison of the United States and Canada or Britain yields interesting results: different institutionalized approaches to medicine yield different rates of diagnoses (Richardson 1989; Armstrong-Hough 2015) and pharmaceutical use (Molstad et al. 2002). However, most of these studies scrutinize countries with similar social and political traditions compared to the diverse arrangements available around the world. Given that there are such diverse institutional arrangements, cultural contexts, and practices of healing even among countries that rely primarily on allopathic biomedicine, focusing on North America, Britain, and other anglophone settings misses some of the most interesting cases. While this book does not focus on institutional differences, such differences profoundly shape the settings in which patients and providers interact and the tools they are able to draw on as they navigate medical encounters.

Similarity amid Difference: Japan and the United States

The United States and Japan are both technologically sophisticated health care systems practicing (primarily) allopathic biomedicine. Both countries have long traditions of evidence-based medicine as well as distinctive folk traditions. In both countries, physicians and other medical professionals participate in an increasingly global community organized around health researchers producing new medical knowledge for global consumption and structured by a grid of national and international guidelines. What can we learn from examining how two wealthy societies that have invested heavily in biomedical approaches to healing treat the same disease?

The United States is widely considered to be both a leader in empirical medical research and a paragon of biomedicalization. American research medicine, often state-subsidized, accounts for a major percentage of new pharmaceuticals and leads the world in the development of new medical procedures (Conrad & Leiter 2004; Conrad 2005). The United States is also a major center of (bio)medicalization, the ever-intensifying social process by which medicine and the medical paradigm become gradually more relevant to laypeople's daily lives (Conrad & Schneider 1992; Clarke et al. 2003). For all these reasons, English-language literature in medical sociology and the sociology of health has focused much of its attention on the United States and, to a lesser extent, the United Kingdom. In the present project, then, the United States works as a reference case in order to relate evidence from another setting to contemporary American sociological theory on medical experience and practice. By including the United States rather than writing only about the burgeoning type 2 diabetes epidemic in Japan, I am able to draw on, critique, and contribute to contemporary medical sociology more effectively.

Like the United States, Japan is an affluent country. It has experienced a significant increase in economic inequality since the beginning of its long recession in 1991, but if anything this has only made Japan's distribution of resources look more like that of the rigidly, unevenly stratified United States. Not only do Japanese doctors practice the same allopathic biomedicine as their colleagues in North America, but Japanese biomedical life sciences research routinely makes contributions to international research medicine (Triendl & Swinbanks 1997). Indeed, the 1987, 2012, 2015, and 2016 Nobel Prizes in Physiology or Medicine went to Japanese nationals, many of whom spent their careers shuttling between Japanese and American research institutions. While most have been basic scientists, one, Shinya Yamanaka, is a Japanese physician-researcher.[5] Japanese research medicine has close ties to American research medicine without being dominated by the American research community.

More importantly, Japanese and American medical communities share the same empirical approach to the production and adjudication of best practices in medicine. Decades of exchange programs, fellowships, and cooperation agreements between Japanese and American universities have brought generations of Japanese physicians to American medical centers on a temporary basis, helping to solidify the sense of shared practice. Yet anthropological studies suggest that certain health practices, narratives, and even beliefs continue to rely on quite distinct medical paradigms and symbolic structures (Ohnuki-Tierney 1984; Norbeck & Lock 1987; Lock 1995; Traphagan 2004; Long 2005). While the standard of medical care available to Japanese and middle-class Americans may be similar, the symbolic content of that medical care can be quite different.

Japan is surprisingly understudied by medical sociologists. During the initial fieldwork for this project, Japan was the second-largest economy in the world (by the time of writing, China surpassed Japan for the number two spot). It is a major producer of medical technology, a major force in global popular culture, and a prime opportunity to examine modernity outside of settings more familiar to U.S. sociology. Yet few medical sociologists study Japan. Instead, Japan has been the purview of medical anthropologists and Japan specialists. In part because Japanese language and cultural competence are perceived to be difficult and time-consuming to acquire, its study has been left to area specialists concentrated in humanistic disciplines. This book approaches Japan with a sociological eye and the hope of contributing to the sociology of health, medical sociology, globalization, and comparative literatures, but also with frequent reference to the work of scholars from other disciplines with a long tradition of attention to Japan.

Obviously, the health systems of the United States and Japan do not only differ on cultural attributes. The institutional contexts of the Japanese health system, a national insurance system in which the vast majority of the population receives health insurance from one of many possible sources, and the U.S. health system, a pluralistic system in which a significant proportion of the population was uninsured at the time of research, are different. While the population of patients and laypeople considered in this book include only those with regular access to medical care, the lack of access to affordable medical care for large numbers of Americans is an undeniable presence in the stories, practices, and assumptions analyzed here. This book is neither about health system differences nor about the impact of such differences on the institutions of medicine in each country. Such a treatment is sorely needed, but I am not the sociologist for the job. Instead, the present work begins from micro-level interviews and observational research, and its focus is trained on the perceptions, experiences, and meaning-making activities of everyday people in two settings.

In the following pages, I aim to examine how patients, providers, and laypeople draw on cultural tool kits to construct different social meanings for diabetes across settings, and how this in turn shapes its management by clinicians, patients, and their families. To extend and globalize theories of medicalization and biomedicalization, I analyze the range of ways in which communities of practice in Japan and the United States explain and respond to diabetes as a biological disruption, as a social problem, and, sometimes, as a spiritual indictment. To accomplish this, I endeavored to start from the experiences, explanations, and habits of people—providers, patients, and families—rather than from the characteristics of institutions.

Two Settings

The arguments presented in this book are grounded in clinic-based fieldwork at multiple sites in Japan and a collection of 359 semistructured interviews with physicians, nurses, co-medicals, patients, and other laypeople in Japan and the United States. The original Japanese interview set included 115 long-form interviews with biomedical professionals (from hospital presidents to endocrinologists to nutritionists) and lay participants (from security guards to retired businessmen to rice farmers). Interviews were conducted in

Japanese, digitally recorded, and transcribed for coding and analysis. A smaller U.S. interview set included 28 long-form interviews, conducted in English, digitally recorded, and transcribed for coding and analysis. More information on this process and its methodological basis in grounded theory is available in the methodological appendix. I supplemented the analysis with an additional 216 health belief and practice interviews with members of the general public from the Japan Multigenerational Interview Project, also described in the methodological appendix.

The initial interview participants in Japan were drawn from two communities: a small town I call Hosekijima[6] and Okayama City, the urban heart of its prefecture. Okayama City is a medium-sized city, home to nearly 700,000 people. Hosekijima, on the other hand, is small by any standard; fewer than 20,000 residents call the hamlet home. Interview participants in the United States were health professionals practicing at a variety of institutions in Durham, North Carolina, a diverse, medium-sized city of 233,000 residents. The final round of interviews were collected from the Kanto and Tohoku regions, including the greater Tokyo area.

Japan and North Carolina are separated by thousands of miles, some fourteen time zones, and two very different languages and lifestyles. There are important differences in the patient mix in these two settings. The average Japanese type 2 diabetes patient is sixty-five years old, while the average American patient is several years younger. Japan's diabetes case registry shows that Japanese patients have a mean BMI of 25 and HbA1c of 7.1 percent (Oishi et al. 2014). Most estimates for American patients are much higher. What all of these communities have in common, though, is an epidemic of type 2 diabetes that is barreling down with unnerving speed. The varieties of response to this epidemic, their origins, and their consequences are the focus of this book.

Organization of the Book

The following chapters, after a discussion of the theoretical framework and central argument in chapter 1, are organized in descending order of imagined social space: world, nation, exam room, and home. Each is a site at which the meaning of the diabetes epidemic is imagined, negotiated, contested, and reimagined.

Chapter 2, "Cavemen Didn't Get Diabetes: American Narratives on the Origins of Type 2 Diabetes," uses the findings of other researchers, a discussion of popular literature on diabetes, and interview data to argue that the dominant American narratives on the origins of the type 2 diabetes epidemic emphasize the universality of risk and rely on the perception that illness arises when one treats the body in ways that are unnatural. The price of modernity, according to this origin story, is stress and the constant temptations of a sedentary lifestyle and unwholesome foods—indulgences that, because they are unnatural, cause harm to the body. Because everyone is imagined to be exposed to risk through indulgence, those that give in to modern temptations and fall victim to so-called lifestyle diseases are implicitly or explicitly cast as morally culpable for their disease.

In chapter 3, "Our Genes Don't Match Your Culture: Japanese Narratives on the Origins of Type 2 Diabetes," I use data gathered from in-depth interviews with clinicians and members of the general public, participant observation, and a brief review of Japanese popular intellectual literature to argue that pervasive Japanese narratives about diabetes emphasize the *particularity* of risk to Japanese bodies and suggest that illness arises from a disconnect between Japanese bodies and non-Japanese food culture. The road to health is a return to an imagined traditional Japanese lifestyle that has been lost to globalization and westernization. Rather than stressing individual responsibility and temptation, dominant Japanese narratives stress a shared struggle against outside forces.

In chapters 4 and 5, I examine clinician strategies for negotiating with patients in order to elicit cooperation and participation in their own self-management. Physicians in both countries switch between different models of the provider-patient relationship as they see fit to the situation. But while American health care providers talk privately about diabetes and patients with diabetes in pessimistic terms, Japanese providers maintain high expectations and hopes for type 2 diabetes outcomes, even in private when they are not cheerleading patients. This difference suggests that clinicians in Japan imagine the origins and inevitable progression of diabetes differently from their peers in the United States—in a way that renders them far more optimistic about patients' futures and more likely to favor lifestyle change. While the preceding chapters rely primarily on interview data, chapter 5 includes participant observation from Japanese exam rooms during eleven months of full-time clinical shadowing. During this time, I shadowed physicians and nurses during both outpatient and inpatient exams at three major health centers, participated in the diabetes education curriculum, attended weekly all-hospital assemblies and medical staff meetings, shadowed dialysis center staff, and shared a group office with the full-time medical doctors on staff.

In chapter 6, "Diabetes at Home: Explanatory Models in Everyday Practice," I use interview data collected from Japanese patients, members of the general public, and health care providers to examine personal explanatory models and illness narratives surrounding type 2 diabetes. Participants articulated a model of health that revolves around the idea of an "ordered" life. In particular, order comes from careful adherence to a classification of time and relies on a clear division of domestic labor. Having a "rhythm" to one's life, and observing regular, unchanging hours for core activities like waking, eating, and bathing were identified as key to a healthy life. But the responsibility for this temporal maintenance falls largely on women: women work to organize the time of loved ones into a healthy, regular rhythm. Men without mothers, wives, sisters, or daughters to take care of them are thus thought to be particularly at risk of illness.

In the conclusion, "Diabetes and Its Discontents," I reflect on the implications of this book for the literatures on global health, globalization, biomedicalization, and the sociology of health.

MICHELLE LAMONT (2000: 251) writes, "Cross-national comparisons reveal otherwise invisible patterns, making national contexts useful sociological laboratories." The cases in this book are bounded by place, and the cultural and institutional settings I examine are embedded in place. In these two national laboratories, we are able to compare the narratives, experiences, and practices of biomedical health professionals, patients, and the public. In doing so, I trace the ways in which context informs—and forms—medical practice in the face of globalization.

CHAPTER ONE

Biomedicalization and Globalization

Biomedicine in Japan

The first time I visited a doctor in Japan, I wondered at the aesthetic differences from my American experiences. I was uneasy in the ill-fitting brown plastic slippers I was asked to exchange for my own shoes before even entering the small primary care clinic's lobby. Were they clean? How was I supposed to walk in them? As I shuffled along behind the nurse on our way to the exam room, one flew off every few steps. I was clumsy and uncomfortable. I was sure that I would rather walk around the clinic barefoot than in slippers that countless patients before me had worn.

I was also perplexed by the nurse's crisp pink uniform and bobby-pinned hat. Compared to the nurses in scrubs that I had grown up with, the clinic nurse looked like she had walked out of another era. I caught myself feeling annoyed. Was it practical for a nurse to wear a dress? Did it have to be pink?

The physician turned out to be a gregarious older man who nodded reassuringly as I described my symptoms and history of upper respiratory infections. After the consultation, I was handed a series of mystifying white packets containing two types of powders, two types of pills, and a small plastic bottle filled with a clear liquid. There was no pharmacy visit; the prescriptions were written and filled in the same room. I was cautioned to wear a mask if I left the house and given instructions to gargle regularly in the future to prevent myself from getting sick again. The last instruction was so foreign that I assumed I had misunderstood, though I would later learn from colleagues that in Japan gargling is widely practiced to prevent colds and influenza.

When I got home, I inspected the packets and their printed dosage instructions. Still a little unnerved by the old-fashioned ambience of the clinic, I looked up each medication on the internet before deciding to follow his instructions. When the search failed to turn up any surprises (and certainly no exotic ingredients), I felt silly for having checked. Biomedicine was biomedicine after all, even in rural Japan.

Japan's relationship with biomedicine goes back centuries. Even before the island nation opened its doors to relatively unfettered trade with the rest of the world, *rangaku* scholars studied Dutch and Russian medical texts and achieved a sophisticated understanding of nascent European medical theory (Jansen 2000, 2002; Jannetta 2007). Despite living in a famously "closed country" under the shogunate, early Japanese physicians studied Chinese and Western medical theory and imported key medical technologies into Japan. Jennerian vaccination, the technique for vaccinating against smallpox using cowpox, was successfully carried out in Japan within approximately fifty years of its discovery half a world away despite the absence of natural cowpox on the Japanese archipelago and the practical difficulties of importing specimens from Europe (Jannetta 2007). By the time Perry "opened" Japan in 1853, Japanese physicians had already carried out sophisticated, large-scale vaccination campaigns using a technique and biological agent imported from Europe.

One reason for this remarkable accomplishment is that physicians were one of the only groups in Tokugawa society permitted by the shogunate to look beyond Japan for practical and theoretical knowledge. Chinese medicine had been practiced in Japan for centuries, but Japanese physicians were pragmatic and ecumenical in their approach to healing. They had access to alternative medical theories and technologies through the work of the *rangaku* scholars. While the esteemed Tokugawa Medical College taught traditional Chinese theory and practice, by the 1600s many Japanese physicians also studied Western medical techniques (Beukers et al. 1991). Doctors who practiced Western style medicine during this period were called *ranpo* (Dutch-method practitioners), gleaning what they could from Dutch or Russian medical texts and anatomical tables (Jannetta 2007: 3).

Consequently, early Japanese physicians developed their own pragmatic, evidence-based approach to medical knowledge distinct from Chinese medicine. Historian Marius B. Jansen describes the first anatomical dissection in Japan, which took place in 1771, writing that "on their way home Sugita and his friends reflected on how shameful it was that they had tried to serve their lords as doctors without first having a true knowledge of the human body" (Jansen 2000: 213). Because Chinese medicine is based on holistic theory, doctors trained in it never opened a body to perform surgery or make anatomical observations. This, combined with social custom that limited contact with the dead to lower-caste Japanese, meant that these highly trained doctors had never seen organs before. The doctors reoriented themselves by committing to empiricism. According to Jansen, "they vowed . . . that thereafter they would seek facts only through experiment" (Jansen 2002: 213).

Later, during Japan's modernization period, the Japanese state built a comprehensive medical education and research system that privileged scientific Western medicine. The first national licensing exam for medical practice in Japan was established in the Medical Act of 1874 and tested examinees on their knowledge of Western medicine, not *kampo* or Chinese medicine (Oberländer 2005). As in the United States, a variety of experiences and practices came under the gaze of public health authorities and the influence of the medical model for the first time, from childbirth (Homei 2006) to nutrition (Bay 2012) to nervous exhaustion (Frühstück 2005) to marriage (through prenuptial health certificates) (Otsubo 2005). As Japan industrialized and embarked on a series of wars and colonial acquisitions, the development, maintenance, and manipulation of Japanese and colonial subjects' bodies became a major focus of the state.[1]

During this period, German medicine was the major international influence on Japanese medicine (Bowers 1979). This was not just true for Japanese medicine; during the late nineteenth century, Germany was the center of emerging international laboratory medicine. In the 1870s and 1880s, American medical education reformers also looked to Germany as a model (Starr 1982). Many of the dramatic educational reforms at Harvard, University of Pennsylvania, and Johns Hopkins medical schools that began to link basic science and clinical practice in the United States took the German model as their inspiration. In Japan, though, the German influence was substantially bolder: in 1870, the Japanese officially and explicitly adopted German medicine, leading to decades of German dominance in its faculties of medicine and in the development of medical terminology. Markers of this long period remain today in the organization of medical faculties and in common terms drawn from the German language, such as レントゲン (*rentogen*), from the German word *Röntgen*, for x-ray.

The postwar period, however, brought increasing contact between the Japanese and American medical research communities and medical education in Japan shifted to emphasize English reading ability in addition to the traditional expectation of German language fluency. Exchange programs brought Japanese physicians and life sciences researchers in contact with major American medical research centers. Joint research programs like the U.S.-Japan Cooperative Medical Science Program, begun in 1965, brought American and Japanese biomedical researchers together to work on health issues affecting lower-income countries in Asia. As the Japanese economy developed at the fastest rate in the world, its own research capacity and pharmaceutical and medical technology industries grew as well. The Japanese market, with its seemingly unlimited potential and hunger for Western products, became a target for American and European pharmaceutical companies, further integrating the content of Japanese biomedical research and practice with the rest of the industrialized world.

Even as Japan's research agenda internationalized, its medical education system remained relatively distinct and, some argued, outdated. Medical education in Japan typically included little critical engagement with research medicine, and the six-year degree program leading to the bachelor and medical doctorate degrees offers little interaction with patients even in the final "clinical" years. Residency programs are shorter in Japan than in the United States, and most postgraduates remain at the school from which they graduated for residency. One American who spent a sabbatical observing general internal medicine training in some of Japan's most prestigious university hospitals in the early 1990s was impressed by the commitment of Japanese medical residents and attendings, but concluded that "the training program in general internal medicine could not be considered modern by U.S. standards" (Tierney 1994). In his description of Japanese academic medicine, he noted residents' preference for "didactic instruction of a non-interactive nature" and discomfort when asked basic questions despite a clear enthusiasm for learning the material, as evidenced by residents' assiduous attendance and note taking.

Nonetheless, by the 1980s and 1990s, physicians in both the United States and Japan were part of an international movement toward evidence-based medicine (EBM). In 1979, a report to the U.S. Congress by the Office of Technology Assessment had argued that only 10 to 20 percent of medical interventions had their foundation in verifiable evidence from controlled trials. While most physicians then and now recognize that a certain degree of their practice is empiric (that is, based on experience rather than scientific evidence), the idea that the vast majority of medical practice was not "scientific medicine" was troubling. And though the originator of the estimate, epidemiologist Dr. Kerr White, himself called it a mere "armchair assessment," the 10 to 20 percent figure was passed around among health care providers and researchers for more than a decade before it was challenged by a new series of retrospective chart reviews in the United States, Britain, and Japan during the 1990s (Gill et al. 1996; Ellis et al. 1995; Tsuruoka et al. 1996).

More than thirty years of efforts to base medical practice in evidence profoundly changed clinical practices around the world. Perhaps inevitably, however, the greatest challenge for evidence-based medicine turned out to be defining the nature of evidence itself. Although the randomized controlled trial was (and is) considered the gold standard for "scientific" evidence of the efficacy of an intervention, the majority of drugs that EBM researchers categorized as "evidenced" had no defined-endpoint randomized controlled trials. These interventions were classified as evidence-based according to *consensus* that the nonexperimental evidence supporting them was sufficient, an approach that raises interesting epistemological questions about how suggestive patterns and experience are transformed into scientific evidence. By including consensus interventions in the "evidence-based" column, Kerr White's armchair assessment proportion could be reversed: around 80 percent of interventions could now be called evidence-based and only around 20 percent unevidenced.

Japanese physicians participated in these international conversations and debates about evidence and practice. In a 1996 reply to a study of evidence-based general practice in the *British Medical Journal*, a group of Japanese medical residents, lecturers, and professors described their inquiry into the proportion of evidence-based medical interventions in Japan. Using a retrospective case note review, the doctors found that 81 percent of the prescription drug choices made by physicians qualified as "evidence-based" because they were either (1) supported by evidence from randomized controlled trials *or* (2) backed up by "convincing non-experimental evidence." (Tsuruoka et al. 1996) This proportion was nearly identical to the proportion of interventions designated "evidence-based" in the original U.K.-based studies (Gill et al. 1996; Sackett et al. 1995) and far greater than previous estimates in the United States (Office of Technology Assessment of the Congress of the United States 1978). Japanese biomedicine was not only based on the same evidence as the rest of the industrialized world, but it relied on that evidence to the same degree as its counterparts in the United States and Britain.

As evidence-based medicine became a global movement, it seemed that medicine could be—would be—science in practice: universal, globally networked, homogenized by shared evidentiary bases, technologies, and guidelines. But does evidence-based medicine mean universal medicine? Does participation in global networks of biomedical knowledge production mean that practices converge? Does integration mean homogenization?

Medicalization

Joint participation in global efforts to build evidence-based and consensus medicine is just one reason we might expect to see increasing similarity between American and Japanese medicine; the two countries have experienced other similar social transformations over the last half-century. In both communities, medicine's sphere of influence expanded rapidly, not only including new disease targets but increasingly focusing attention on health itself through the articulation of categories of risk, states of pre-illness, and states of health that could be optimized through intervention. That is, Japanese and American societies have both undergone a series of social changes that have made biomedical approaches to managing and preserving life increasingly more central to daily life.

Medicalization, the process by which biomedicine and the biomedical paradigm become more relevant to social life, has been central to the transformation of medicine as a social institution in the United States, Japan, and around the world (Conrad 2005). Over the course of the twentieth century, a host of experiences and problems came under the purview of American medicine, including childbirth, alcohol and drug dependency, chronic unhappiness, childhood behavioral problems, sexual difficulties, and obesity. Many of these were previously framed as personal problems, or as moral or social problems managed by other social institutions such as the church, the family, or even the justice system.

Even as practices in Japan remained different from those in North America throughout the twentieth century, Japan was no stranger to medicalization or the growth of pharmaceutical solutions. By 1976, Japan's per capita pharmaceutical consumption by value was among the highest in the world, approximately tying the United States (WHO 2004).[2] Thanks to a near-universal health insurance system, Japanese citizens have access to inexpensive health care, which they utilize enthusiastically: the average Japanese patient is seen by a physician more than thirteen times per year, tied with South Korea for the highest number of annual visits in the OECD.[3] Much like in the United States, Japanese physicians enjoy high social status, significant political influence, and a role as trusted and impartial experts in judicial proceedings and everyday life. Unlike in the United States, the medical profession in Japan has largely kept medical authority for itself, successfully preventing nursing professionals, co-medicals, or professional administrators and executives from expanding into their domain. This has remained possible in part because, by law, all Japanese medical facilities must be owned and managed by physicians and because physicians form a large portion of the influential governmental committee that assigns all medical procedures, supplies, and medications their point value in the national health insurance system.

The best measure of medicalization, though, is the degree to which previously nonmedical issues and problems are reframed as within the purview of modern medicine. Here, too, Japan proves to be one of the most medicalized societies in the world: alcoholism, menopause, and senility all shifted from being thought of as social problems or social transformations to issues within the purview of medicine over the course of the twentieth century. Medicalization of diseases and disorders like Hansen's disease and metabolic syndrome has reduced, though certainly not eliminated, the stigma of some conditions that would previously have reduced their victims to social pariahs.

As in the United States, new states of illness continue to be produced and marketed in Japan. In one of the most recent examples of this process, the medical associations that advise the insurance point system on which all medical care reimbursement is based recognized excessive underarm sweat as a disease. As a recent spring heated up, GlaxoSmithKline papered Tokyo's crowded subway cars with advertisements notifying potential patients that excessive sweating was now known to be a disease, that they could consult with their doctor about it, and that their national insurance would cover their treatment. Packed-in passengers spend their steamy commutes reading overhead signs urging, "Please don't agonize alone. You can ask your doctor about it." Alternatively, finer print reads, you can visit the website or call to receive a manual with advice about controlling embarrassing perspiration.

One important difference in the course of medicalization in Japan is the prominence and popularity of traditional medicines. Since 1967, the national health insurance system has covered certain *kampo* herbal medicines and procedures — but only if prescribed by a licensed biomedical physician. Approximately 2 percent of all prescriptions written by biomedical physicians in Japan are for *kampo* drugs and 80 percent of doctors prescribe *kampo* (Fuyuno 2011). Medical anthropologists have long noted that practitioners and consumers of traditional medicines in Japan embrace the approach and language of biomedicine in their use of Chinese medicine or herbal traditions. Margaret Lock observed that Japanese practice of traditional East Asian medicine in the 1970s "did not usually operate within an integrated approach to health and illness or to mind and body" as one might assume, but rather that "practitioners appeared to be engaged in an attempt to remove physical symptoms in a fashion reminiscent of that of most biomedical physicians, although their tools were those of traditional medicine" (Lock 1980: v–vi). Japan's health care system is pluralistic, but the biomedical paradigm and evidence-based adjudication of knowledge are hegemonic even outside the boundaries of biomedicine.

Importantly, the boundaries and targets of medicalization in Japan and the United States also differ. While medicalization scholars in the United

States have given much attention to the far-reaching medicalization of so-cial problems through psychiatry and psychopharmaceutical market cre-ation, psychiatry and its consumables are neither as prevalent nor as differentiated in Japan as in the United States. Even as attention deficit dis-orders, general anxiety disorders, and mood disorders proliferate in the United States, psychological states are differently medicalized—and typically less medicated—in Japan. In the global market for pharmaceuticals, for ex-ample, while the United States consumes more ADHD medications than would be expected based on the size of its GDP, Japan consumes far fewer ADHD drugs than would be expected (Scheffler et al. 2007; Armstrong-Hough 2018). And while per capita antidepressant consumption is on the rise in Japan, it remains low compared to the United States (Nakagawa et al. 2007). In diagnosis, treatment, and social recognition of medicalized mental distress, Japan's path has been different from the United States.

This is not for lack of opportunity—indeed, potential targets for medi-calization proliferate in contemporary Japanese society. Japanese children and adolescents are famously under enormous educational pressure, prob-lems of adjustment are common, and the long-term consequences of fail-ure to perform academically from an early age in an exam-based system are grave. Rates of suicide among Japanese adolescents are about twice as high as in the United States. *Hikikomori*, a phenomenon wherein adoles-cents or young adults completely withdraw from all social life by refusing to leave their closed rooms for months, years, or decades at a time, receives significant attention from the media and in popular culture. Japan's adult male suicide rate ranks in the top ten highest in the world, and its adult female suicide rate is second highest in the world by some measures; the combined suicide rate for both genders is roughly double that of the United States (Yoshioka et al. 2010). In recent years, Ministry of Health, Labor, and Welfare surveys have shown that nearly a quarter of Japanese young women in their twenties are clinically underweight, and many underweight women continue to diet, suggesting that eating disorders are more common in Japan than widely assumed.

Yet unhappiness, anxiety, suicide, *hikikomori*, and excessive dieting are all framed first as social issues in Japan, not medical issues. Efforts to reduce suicide have focused on reforming life insurance policy practices and even changing the physical environment to make it physically more difficult to commit suicide in public, rather than expanding health screening for major depressive disorder, the mood disorder implicated in a significant propor-tion of suicides (Duignan 2012). Marketing attempts for antidepressants portray depression as a temporary rather than chronic state: "a cold of the soul" (*kokoro no kaze*), to translate the enormously influential pharmaceutical campaign that popularized selective serotonin reuptake inhibitors. *Hikikomori* may worry family and social workers, but it is unlikely a physician or psychiatrist will be consulted. Though eating disorders are beginning to receive more attention, they are often framed as problems of excess rather than as mental illnesses. While medicalization has progressed in Japan, its colonies are not identical to those of American medicine.

Pharmaceuticalization

By the 2000s, the expansion of the biomedical paradigm into American daily life was increasingly driven by the allure of pharmaceutical solutions and enhancements. Scholars theorized a parallel process, pharmaceuticalization, variously defined as "the transformation of human conditions, capacities, or capabilities into pharmaceutical matters for treatment or enhancement" (Williams et al. 2009; see also Williams et al. 2011) and "the process by which social, behavioural, or bodily conditions are treated or deemed to be in need of treatment, with medical drugs by doctors or patients" (Abraham 2009). Medicalization, marketing of pharmaceutical products for both established and emerging medicalized conditions, and popular assumptions that pharmaceutical solutions epitomize medical progress contributed to the growing centrality of pharmaceuticals even as therapeutically significant innovations in the pharmaceutical industry declined (Abraham 2010).

Although pharmaceuticalization and medicalization interrelate, they are distinct phenomena. The expansion of reliance on pharmaceuticals does not demand medicalization, because drugs may be increasingly applied to treat established medical conditions (Abraham 2010). Similarly, John Abraham argues, pharmaceuticalization may occur independent of medicalization when "the medical profession is by-passed in pharmaceutical choice, purchase and use" (2010: 605), such as when consumers seek drugs over-the-counter without consulting medical gatekeepers. While this latter distinction depends on a rather narrow conceptualization of medicalization as the expansion of the medical profession, rather than as the expansion of biomedical approaches to managing life, the separation of medicalization and pharmaceuticalization into distinct axes is an important conceptual step for generalizing these theories to other settings. In Japan, as in the United States, medicalization in the twentieth century was accompanied by the rise of a powerful pharmaceutical industry and enthusiastic consumption of pharmaceutical products. Japanese physicians often point out that medical consumers in Japan do not feel that their complaint has been addressed if they are not prescribed a drug, and the pharmaceuticalization of risk has produced large numbers of "the subjectively healthy but highly medicated" (Greene 2007). Yet while pharmaceuticalization has been associated with a diminished role of the medical profession in the United States, this is not necessarily the case in Japan.

Sociologists and anthropologists have argued that the dominant theoretical frame used to understand pharmaceuticalization in sociology is limited by its emphasis on "western" settings. Bell and Figert (2012) point out that, in sociology, "the majority of scholarship has investigated pharmaceuticalization as a modern process and conceptualized it in modern terms" (781). The concept of biomedicalization, on the other hand, with its origins in postmodern theory, can be used to illuminate postmodern processes.

Biomedicalization

Over the last 15 years, theories of biomedicalization have generated new perspectives on the processes transforming biomedicine and expanding its domain beyond illness to health itself. What distinguishes biomedicalization from preceding (and still ongoing) medicalization is its scope, scale, and intensity. Biomedicalization widens the scope of biomedical intervention from pathology to life itself, scales up biomedicine as an institution through increasingly complex and dense economic relations, and intensifies the biomedical gaze through technoscientific modes of measuring health and a shift to individualizing genetic etiologies and solutions. In their defining survey of biomedicalization, Clarke et al. (2003) identified five broad processes of biomedicalization: privatization and commodification, risk and surveillance, expanding technoscientific practices, the production and distribution of knowledge, and transformations of bodies and subjectivities.

Although most empirical work engaging with the biomedicalization framework is still U.S.-based, biomedicalization is not confined to North America. Clarke and her colleagues argue that "these transformations of medical care and of life itself are, of course, increasingly exported and (re)-modeled as well as being produced elsewhere" and call for more empirical work on medicalization and biomedicalization outside the U.S. context (Clarke et al. 2010: 32). The present work is, in part, a response to that call. Japan and the United States, with their long but varied histories of empirical biomedicine and medicalization, make excellent comparative cases for understanding how biomedicalization interacts with its contexts.

Just as medicalization played a role in the development of Japanese medicine in ways that sometimes mirror and sometimes contradict American medicalization patterns, biomedicalization is also emerging as a central process of social change in contemporary Japan—but not always in the ways we might expect based on the North American experience. On the one hand, biomedicalization has clearly advanced in Japan along several of the dimensions articulated in Clarke et al.'s original framework (2003, 2010). On the other hand, the targets and consequences of biomedicalization in Japan differ from those in the United States. Because almost all work on biomedicalization has focused on North America and readers are less likely to be familiar with Japan, it is worthwhile to mention a few of these *similarities in process* alongside their *differences in target and consequences*. I briefly examine three dimensions here: the intensifying focus on health and states of pre-illness, growing emphasis on surveillance and risk, and deepening technoscientization in health practices.

Intensifying Focus on Health and Pre-illness

By the beginning of the twenty-first century, the focus on health intensified and states of *pre*-illness or *potential* illness were demarcated, denormalized, and increasingly managed through biomedical intervention in Japan. Not surprisingly, given the country's demographic profile, particular care is expended toward the maintenance of healthy aging bodies. An early morning walk through most urban neighborhood parks in Tokyo, for example, is likely to encounter elderly residents practicing *rajio taisou* ("radio exercise") in groups, a series of calisthenics narrated on the radio each morning. Daytime television includes scheduled breaks for stretching and range-of-motion exercises; students from a Tokyo-based physical education university lead viewers through the movements, which are designed to be done easily within the narrow confines of Japanese homes and demonstrated with modifications for people whose age or impairment make it difficult to fully move through the combinations.

Japanese mass media also enthusiastically educate their public about new states of pre-illness that responsible consumers should be aware of and, if necessary, manage. Like in the United States, health is a common subject of morning and daytime news programs. Unlike in the United States, flashy medical talk shows are also part of primetime network television.[4] In one popular primetime show, the mega-celebrity host dons an oversized doctor costume resembling pajamas and introduces the audience to a medical problem they probably didn't know they had: eyes damaged by UV rays, preskin cancer, frequent urination, visceral fat, prediabetes, hardening arteries as a result of insufficient professional dental care, and so on. The emphasis of the show is on subclinical pathologies or abnormalities that may eventually develop into more serious conditions. A series of short vignettes about people who have these problems is shown, followed by a panel of minor celebrities who discuss and make self-deprecating jokes. Next, a serious-faced guest doctor in a white coat details the etiology, prognosis, and screening options for the condition, and the celebrity panel's own test results are shared. The doctor describes research showing how they can improve their results through particular behavior changes, diet modifications, exercises, or medical procedures. This research is then demonstrated as the show follows a panel member or guest patient who diligently makes the changes to daily life recommended by the doctor. At the end, their "before" and "after" test results are compared, confirming the efficacy of these daily behavioral changes. Disease is depicted as a long, inevitable road, with a series of pre-illness stages that can (and should) be identified and managed by putting biomedical knowledge into practice in one's daily life.

The emphasis on pre-illness is particularly intense for those at risk of type 2 diabetes. A widely cited meta-analysis of the effect of lifestyle education intervention on progression from impaired glucose tolerance (IGT) to diabetes found that such interventions reduce one-year incidence of diabetes by 50 percent (Yamaoka & Tango 2005). In Japan, a trial testing the effect of lifestyle intervention on progression from IGT to diabetes among men found a 67 percent reduction of cumulative four-year incidence of diabetes (Kosaka, Noda, & Kuzuya 2005). The lifestyle intervention involved repetition of detailed lifestyle advice during hospital visits every two to four months; men in the control arm merely received advice to decrease their meal size, increase physical activity, and aim for a lower BMI during hospital visits every six months (Kosaka, Noda, & Kuzuya 2005). Another intervention that provided a diabetes-education-style group curriculum to patients with IGT reduced progression to diabetes by 50 percent over three years (Sakane et al. 2011). These trials suggested that focusing biomedical resources on preillness risk groups could yield dramatic public health benefits.

By the early 2000s, endocrinologists in both the United States and Japan were considering questions about the extent to which prediabetes states should be medicalized—and medicated (Simpson, Shaw, & Zimmet 2003). What of pharmacotherapy for the "otherwise well"? Though there was convincing evidence that lifestyle intervention could slow progression to diabetes mellitus (DM) by 50 percent or more, such interventions were difficult to apply and sustain in everyday practice (Simpson, Shaw, & Zimmet 2003). Lifestyle change is harder than medication; compared to medication, adherence to lifestyle interventions is poor (Peyrot et al. 2005). Now doctors asked: should IGT be treated with pharmacotherapy to prevent progression to DM?

In the United States, risk factors have gradually expanded into pre-disease states that patients and providers liken to illness; nearly half of American adults are diagnosed and treated for risk-based conditions (Kreiner & Hunt 2014). In Japan, similarly, it is common for patients to be diagnosed with IGT years before developing type 2 diabetes or even prediabetes. Patients' IGT is labeled, quantified, monitored, and actively managed. For the patient, this is its own diagnosis. Some interview respondents initially volunteered that they had diabetes themselves, then clarified that their glucose tolerance was impaired, though not within the clinical threshold for diabetes (or even prediabetes, in some cases). They did not have diabetes—but they *anticipated* having diabetes, they were preparing to have diabetes, and this state of pre-illness was already a part of their identity. I examine these pre-illness identities in more detail in chapter 6, "Diabetes at Home."

Risk and Surveillance

Japanese society also evidences a growing emphasis on surveillance and risk similar to what biomedicalization scholars have noted in U.S. contexts. In part due to public health education efforts (Udagawa, Miyoshi, & Yoshiike 2008) and in part due to public anxiety over the future of Japan's health care system as the population ages, most consumers of mass media are able to articulate remarkably detailed risk profiles for chronic disease. In interviews with members of the general public for this book, Japanese participants frequently professed nervousness that they might miss or forget a risk factor that they were supposed to know, as if the interview were a pop quiz. Other respondents ticked risk factors and the categories of people they were thought to most affect with such fluidity that one had the impression they had heard the risk categories hundreds of times in the same order.

The proliferation of risk *surveillance* in Japan has likewise been extraordinary. Like the United States, the Japanese government collects reams of data on the nation's health status and produces estimates for change in the future. Medical variety shows like those mentioned above train viewers to self-monitor by identifying their own risk level and self-screening for early indicators of disease. Workplace screening programs and workplace demands for annual or biannual physical exams mean that many working Japanese not only have access to health evaluations but the *obligation* to be evaluated. Many of these screening programs are conducted semipublicly, at workplaces, which may further reinforce the social pressure to self-monitor and preemptively manage risk.

However, the production of risk and modes of surveillance are often constituted differently in Japan. As I discuss in chapters 3 and 4, the social production of risk categories relies on underlying narratives about natural and unnatural ways of living that differ between the United States and Japan. While U.S. narratives about the origins of Americans' risk for type 2 diabetes tell a story of mismatch between bodies evolved in a universally shared past and a modern environment full of temptation, Japanese narratives tell a story of mismatch between bodies evolved in a particular and separate past and a modern environment full of foreign, racialized foods and practices. Chapter 2, "Cavemen Didn't Get Diabetes," examines the production of risk narratives for diabetes in the United States, while chapter 3, "Our Genes Don't Match Your Culture," examines the production of these narratives in Japan.

Modes of surveillance also differ. In Japan, the three social institutions that organize almost all productive and reproductive life are also the main sites of risk surveillance and management: education, work, and family. In educational and work institutions, screening for disease, pre-disease, and risk is built into individuals' obligation to the institution itself. Annual checkups, screenings, and preventative interventions are conducted on site at schools or workplaces. Students and workers who skip these events (this author included) may escape requirements like the dreaded chest x-ray for TB screening for a year or two, but eventually the long arm of their institution's bureaucracy will reach out to compel participation. Non-Japanese workers are often surprised by how coercive the screening requirements are in Japan compared to home countries and by how little choice they have in how the screening is to take place.

But it is within the domestic sphere that some of the most interesting surveillance and risk management occurs. The primetime medical variety show mentioned above, for example, is explicitly designed to give its viewers medical knowledge they can put into practice *in the home*: its name, *"Takeshi no kenko entateinmento! Minna no katei no igaku"* translates to

"Takeshi's health entertainment! Home medical study for everyone." In the home, women are deputized to monitor and manage the health of the men in their household. Chapter Six, "Diabetes at Home," examines in details the ways in which risk is perceived and managed within the rigidly gendered domestic sphere. Similarly, the high expectations Japanese clinicians have of patients' ability to self-manage their diabetes (chapter 5) are premised on the assumption that the home is an ordered space managed by female family members who can be trusted to manage the patient's behavior change.

Technoscientization

Finally, the technoscientization of health practice has progressed in Japan as in the United States, perhaps more evenly than in the United States. Even as patients are encouraged to carefully monitor and document their own food consumption, activity levels, and physical well-being, success is measured with laboratory tests. Perhaps because the Japanese fee schedule for medical reimbursement incentivizes laboratory tests, which require little physician time, Japanese physicians order more laboratory and diagnostic tests than their international peers and there are more diagnostic imaging machines per capita in Japan than in the United States (Ikegami & Campbell 1995). As a result, as in the United States, checkups revolve around technical results that often represent surrogate outcomes rather than outcomes that are immediately relevant to patients' quality of life (Yudkin, Lipska, & Montori 2011)—progress or failure is measured by HbA1c levels, triglycerides, forced expiratory volume, and so on.

Even in Beat Takeshi's show, which emphasizes everyday behaviors and self-maintenance and health improvement activities that can be undertaken in the comfort of one's own home, the patient's improved sense of well-being is *not* the mark of a successful intervention. Rather, the change in their quantifiable results on a variety of laboratory tests is the mark of success. Guests' precise scores—blood glucose, HbA1c, blood pressure, proportion of fat in their liver, and so on—are displayed over their faces as they react to the good news with smiles and relief.

Theories of biomedicalization emphasize transformations and movement—for this reason, biomedicalization theory is flexible and responsive to new knowledge. But examinations of the phenomenon in North America may mistake it for a homogenizing, rationalizing social process. Comparing Japan to the United States reminds us that transformations of biomedical knowledge, practice, and co-optation do not follow a set path in every context. Rather, the very dynamism of biomedicalization interacts with its contexts to create myriad possibilities and probabilities. If we look away from the familiar U.S. context, we see biomedicalization processes re-inscribing different social values and assumptions into social practice than in North America.

Biomedicalization, Globalization, and the Problem of the Local

One of the reasons medicine is such an interesting subject for social scientists is that it is a privileged area of knowledge, a set of beliefs and practices made sacrosanct by their close relationship to empirical science. In many set-tings, biomedicine is treated as if it is above tradition, belief, and culture—a value-free arbiter of truth rather than a fundamentally social practice. This makes medicine a fascinating and challenging subject for social scientists.

This attribute also makes it easy to assume that, with globalization, biomedicine will eventually and inevitably achieve a global homogeneity in content: the local will be erased as rationalization progresses. As biomedi-calization travels transnationally, as biomedicine becomes an increasingly global enterprise, what becomes of the local? It is tempting to see "global" processes like biomedicalization as homogenizing influences that will in-evitably overpower difference and "local" processes and transformations as particularistic holdouts against the pressures of rationalization.

As globalization scholars have observed, however, when we approach the global and the local as a binary in this way, both become homogenizing frames. The global becomes a looming monolith; the local is flattened into an essentializing series of unchanging, unvaried practices and orientations. The variety of locals in a single community is erased: differences and dis-agreements are folded into one another and hidden from view by the aggre-gate identity. And with the erasure of difference and disagreement within communities, their dynamism, too, is erased: the creative manipulation of tropes, the repositioning of identities, the reframing of origin narratives, the shifts in moral evaluations. In the global-local binary, the local is rendered a strangely tame, eerily unvaried landscape.

Perhaps no industrialized country or culture has been so thoroughly localized (and Orientalized) by twentieth-century globalization discourse as Japan. Its postwar economic ascent and integration into the global economy only seemed to further establish Japanese society as a modernity apart, an alternative dimension with unique business customs rooted in supposedly ancient codes and modes of social organization. In this caricature of Japan,

Japanese people become mere ciphers empowered only to carry out stylized repetitions of an imagined past: samurai values in business, geisha tropes in gender relations, Confucian principles in education.

This is a strange thing to believe about the citizens of one of the largest economies in the world, a major production site for global popular culture, and a dizzyingly differentiated consumer market. Japanese society, reassembled and reimagined from the ruins of World War II, which incinerated its urban landscapes and cost the emperor's divinity, is nothing if not dynamic. Yet the claim that Japan and the Japanese "way" (of business, of studying, of marriage, of eating, of playing) are singular proliferates. And the claim that this "way" is unchanging—rooted in an ancient, exotic past—seems to re-surface every time something important has demonstrably changed.

I am eager to avoid the intellectual trap that the homogenizing frames of the global-local binary set for us, particularly in writing about Japan. But doing so requires great care, not only in describing the nature of globaliza-tion itself but also in theorizing biomedicalization as a series of globalizing social processes. How are we to understand the process by which medical-ization and biomedicalization inscribe different assumptions into social prac-tice in different contexts without reducing the local to a frozen caricature? How does a globalizing process produce such different results in different places, if not because of the resistance and reconfigurations wrought by per-sistent locals?

I argue that in both the United States and Japan, there is evidence of an intensifying prerogative for "controlling, managing, engineering, reshaping, modulating" humans' vital capacities: what Nikolas Rose calls "the politics of life itself" (2007a). Patients are urged to be active and responsible consum-ers of medicine. Yet, as I've described above, the targets, sites, and conse-quences of this prerogative for active and responsible consumption vary between the United States and Japan, leaving open the possibility that they are inscribed with specific expectations and values in each place. And as I've described above and in the introduction, the biomedical responses to type 2 diabetes—from conventions of practice to intervention choices—also vary between the United States and Japan.

I theorize biomedicalization as a series of social transformations through which the practice of everyday life and the practice of medicine are power-fully connected to the production of purportedly universal (and thus "true") knowledge through technoscience. I argue that the practice of everyday life is not simply colonized by biomedicine or biomedical ways of thinking about the world; the practice of everyday life interacts with, reframes, and reshapes technoscientific biomedicine in its various contexts to a variety of ends. The framing and contours of biomedicine thus depend on its contexts, and bio-medicalization is not a vehicle for specific content, practices, or values.

Biomedicalization, in this view, is a collection of technologies of rationale, which can be used to reinscribe and reify multiple possible narratives about the nature of the body with multiple possible implied social values and mul-tiple possible social interpretations. In other words, biomedicalization is a process through which certain sources of legitimacy are strengthened while others are shunted aside, but these new sources of legitimacy can be used to a variety of social ends.

Such transformations in legitimacy and legitimating rationales, of course, have consequences for power. In the United States, for example, it is clear that biomedicalization has contributed to the inscription of neoliberal claims about human nature and individual responsibility into our very bodies. The shadows of these claims are evident in the discourse on risk and responsi-bility examined in the U.S. chapters of this book. But because these trans-formations rely on existing narratives in existing social contexts, their production of new content always occurs with reference to existing, often intuitive narratives. We will, for example, see different claims about nature and responsibility in the chapters examining Japan than in those examining the United States.

It is here that culture enters. I treat culture as a resource, following soci-ologists like Ann Swidler and Jeffrey Alexander. To analyze the role of cul-ture in biomedicine and biomedicalization, I start from Swidler's classic cultural tool kit approach. Swidler rejects previous models of culture that posit that culture shapes action by supplying the values toward which action is directed. Turning away from a value-oriented explanation of culture's effect on action, Swidler argues that culture shapes action independent of values by shaping the cultural tool kits ("habits, skills, and styles") from which people build strategies of action (Swidler 1986: 273). Culture provides the resources from which people construct action.

Like all tool kits, culture both constrains and facilitates creative transfor-mation. Culture does not determine ends but rather equips individuals with the narrative, normative, and symbolic means through which ends are pursued. My approach is to treat culture as resources that can be drawn on, curated, applied, and refashioned by their users. These resources can vary both between and within communities.

I argue that both biomedicalization and the everyday practice of biomed-icine rest on relatively widely shared narratives within communities. These narratives and narrative fragments are accessed selectively and deployed with creativity and contradiction by members of collectives. The "local" is not an internally homogenous, externally particular site colonized by the universal forces of science, globalization, and biomedicalization. Rather, the "local" is a dynamic site of contradictory agendas, contestations, and assumptions where global legitimating rationales are deployed in interaction with elements of locally available cultural tool kits to achieve local ends.

Therefore, there is no predetermined path or preordained site of power accumulation or social value as biomedicalization progresses. Further, the transformations we call biomedicalization are necessarily inflected and informed by their sociocultural context through what is available and selected from the tool kit, how it is deployed, and who/what its target is. For example, in chapter 3, I argue that "things medical" are not only the source material for popular depictions of Japanese identity. Popular depictions of Japanese identity shape and even create "things medical" in the Japanese context.

Rather than emphasizing the contrast between purportedly universal biomedical models and local models, I hope to emphasize that biomedicine itself is a diverse social enterprise and that a plurality of explanatory models are not only available but thriving within its boundaries. Biomedicine is persistently plural because clinical encounters require both patients and providers to construct narratives from cultural materials. For all their universalizing and rationalizing pretentions, biomedicine and biomedicalization have multiple presents—and, likely, multiple futures.

Biomedicalization and the Production of Difference in Responses to Type 2 Diabetes

In his classic study of medical cultures in Taiwan, Arthur Kleinman examined the process by which individuals develop different explanatory models of healing, arguing that "cultural context" influences a population's general beliefs about health and healing, which in turn shape the "health care system" in important ways. "Health care system" is in quotation marks here because Kleinman used the term to refer to the complex social system of healing, not simply the political economy of medicine. This health care system, in turn, supports explanatory models, which people construct in response to specific disease or illness episodes.[5] Importantly, Kleinman writes that "the metaphors used to articulate both patient and practitioner explanatory models disclose substantial cultural patterning" (Kleinman 1981: 107).

What Kleinman calls a society's "health care system" resembles Swidler's cultural tool kit. In the face of illness, patients creatively construct explanations and strategies of action from the tool kit that is available to them, which results in cultural patterning but certainly not homogeneity. Throughout this book, I examine these patterned differences in explanatory models and narratives about the origins of type 2 diabetes by focusing on three relatively straightforward questions: What are appropriate and healthy uses of the body? Who exercises legitimate medical authority, and how? Finally, who takes responsibility for individual health?

As ways of thinking about the body, authority, and responsibility in health contexts diverge, so do the characters of biomedicine and biomedicalization in each context. In the United States, biomedical models often align with a capitalist ethic of productivity and responsibility, and the individual is continually reinscribed as the primary category of being and object of medicine. In Japan, biomedical models often align instead with discourses of nationhood, membership in a unique racial-cultural community, and gendered domestic labor. Biomedical discourses on the possibility of wellness and the risk of illness exist within the framework of the family and the community, not the individual.

Some literature on medicalization and biomedicalization has suggested that the increasing status of biomedicine acts on, influences, or even colonizes local models of health, illness, and healing. I propose that local models instead colonize biomedicine. The character of biomedicine in any context, including at elite medical centers in the United States, is profoundly shaped by pervasive narratives about the nature of the body, authority, and responsibility. These underlying models influence provider behavior as much as patient behavior.

Explanatory models, built from local narrative materials, work on provider and patient behavior by framing what makes intuitive "sense." At the same time, globalization profoundly affects the language in which these models are expressed. Japanese laypeople hypothesizing about the origins of diabetes, for example, frequently refer to evolution, genetics, and scientific biomedicine to support their narrative. American lay narratives about the origins of diabetes also rely on quasi-scientific claims about evolution and human natural history. But even while relying on shared global, cosmopolitan references to explain illness, Japanese and Americans use them to construct different narratives about the causes, treatment, and appropriate prevention of diabetes.

Culture should not be used as a master explanatory device for difference. As I have discussed elsewhere in this chapter, reliance on culture as an explanatory device almost necessarily produces essentialist and homogenizing accounts of culture, while cloaking less convenient sources of difference or disparity. If attention to culture is to elucidate rather than obscure, we must pay attention to the ways in which culture is applied as a resource. In this monograph, I examine the practice of culture by real people to characterize, make sense of, and produce (and rationalize) responses to the epidemic of type 2 diabetes in their respective settings.

This use of shared biomedical language to articulate very different visions of the diabetes epidemic and its best management is a *technology of rationale*. Because biomedicine enjoys such high status in both societies, biomedical language is an important source of legitimation for these narratives and explanatory models. As these technologies of rationale are dispersed by globalization, we see rapid convergence in some aspects of the language professionals (and eventually laypeople) use to articulate the etiology and nature of diabetes. The vocabulary of biomedical stories is increasingly shared. And yet the stories themselves—of the origins of diabetes in the population, etiology in the individual, and best management—remain distinct. The following chapters examine, compare, and analyze the origins and consequences of these stories that use such similar language and yet reach such different conclusions.

Several of the chapters that follow explore how people use claims about culture to explain, understand, come to terms with, and respond to the ascendance of type 2 diabetes. When respondents in chapter 3 echo dated tropes in their discussions of the origins of diabetes in Japan, the pervasive claim that Japanese culture is unique is not my analysis. Rather, it is the object of my analysis. Considering the ways in which ordinary people curate and apply tropes about being Japanese, being American, or being a modern human to explain the rise of diabetes deepens our understanding of how biomedicalization is transformed even as it transforms its setting. I caution the reader that these essentialist tropes are tools of convenience, drawn on when they are useful for making sense of illness to oneself or to a patient, not necessarily closely held ideologies.

CHAPTER TWO

Cavemen Didn't Get Diabetes

American Narratives about the Origins of Type 2 Diabetes

Sofie Loftis, an athletic blonde in her midthirties, told me she doesn't look the part. Though a publicist for a professional sports team sponsored by a pharmaceutical company known for its oral and injectable antidiabetics, she avoids mentioning her polycystic ovary syndrome (PCOS)-related type 2 diabetes to strangers. Most people, she has learned, do not take the news gracefully. Surprised, they blurt out objections: "But you're so fit!" A slim, overachieving endurance athlete who once walked for most of a day with an excruciating knee injury rather than permit a brace to ruin the line of her dress, Sofie's social identity revolves around extraordinary discipline. She is not the sort of person Americans think is supposed to get diabetes.

This chapter introduces American discourse on the origins of the diabetes epidemic. I argue that this discourse emphasizes universal risk and rests on pervasive perceptions that illness arises when one treats the body in ways that are "unnatural." Popular accounts portray the road to health as a life disciplined by natural rhythms, in contrast to the stress- and temptation-filled lives that are possible in modern America. Popular understanding of diabetes risk rests largely on what anthropologist Leslie Aiello and biologist Marlene Zuk have memorably labeled "paleofantasy," the widely accepted but empirically suspect just-so stories of evolutionary history that pervade American popular culture. This powerful narrative on the origins of the type 2 diabetes epidemic emphasizes universality of diabetes risk to all citizens of modernity, alongside the idea that groups associated with certain lifestyles *put themselves* at higher risk by behaving in evolutionarily unprecedented or unwise ways. Americans strongly associate diabetes with obesity, and this association is burdened with moralistic overtones that overshadow the socioeconomic and genetic patterning of diabetes risk. Even health care providers draw on this narrative, speaking in interviews of "my-fault diabetes," informally observed correlations between "type B personalities" and diabetes, and the emotional work of fairly treating patients with illness that arose at least in part from their "own" behavior.

In this chapter, I synthesize findings from the various literatures on patient models of type 2 diabetes, analysis of popular discourse in the popular literature on diabetes, and interviews with American health providers and members of the general public. I conclude with a discussion of the alternative narratives to paleofantasy and blame that can be found in African American guides to diabetes management. In these materials, choice is situated within a broader social context that is understood to powerfully shape the lifestyle that puts African Americans at higher risk for illness. This narrative is closer to pervasive Japanese explanations of the type 2 diabetes epidemic covered in the next chapter than to the narratives that dominate other American health materials.

This chapter deals only peripherally with individual patients' ideas about what in their personal experience precipitated the onset of type 2 diabetes. Much excellent work has already been done on the personal explanatory models of American patients with type 2 diabetes (Borovoy & Hine 2008; Chesla et al. 2000, 2009; Ferzacca 2000; Lange & Piette 2006; Loewe & Freeman 2000; Hampson et al. 1990, 1995, 1997; Glasgow et al. 1997; Poss & Jezewski 2002; Schoenberg et al. 2005; Mercado-Martinez & Ramos-Herrera 2002). However, defining the materials from which American providers and patients piece together their approach to diabetes requires examination of wider understandings and stories about *why the type 2 diabetes epidemic is growing in the United States*. Answers to the questions "Why do you think you got diabetes at the time that you did?" and "Why do you think diabetes rates are rising in this country?" can be very different. The wider context in which patients creatively construct their explanatory models is key to understanding those models because explanatory models exist and are only interpretable within the context of a complex social system of healing. Explanatory models are constructed by individuals in response to a specific disease or illness episode, but they are patterned in important ways by the wider sociocultural context.

Modernity and Risk

Anthropologists have found that patients tend to identify social, economic, or relational factors when describing the origins of their own diabetes (Schoenberg et al. 2005; Mercado-Martinez & Ramos-Herrera 2002). While lay articulations of the origins of diabetes overlap with biomedical models, especially in the language in which they are presented, they also embrace the influence of the wider social context. Many patients point to "changing life circumstances" as the fundamental cause of their own diabetes (Schoenberg et al. 2005; Poss & Jezewski 2002; Hunt et al. 1998). In particular, personal models of diabetes etiology in U.S. populations emphasize the central role of stress (Schoenberg et al. 2005; Loewe & Freeman 2000; Cohen et al. 1994). One anthropological examination of the diabetes explanatory models of eighty American patients from a diverse sampling of backgrounds found that across all ethnic groups the majority of American patients identified stress, in one form or another, as the origin of their diabetes (Schoenberg et al. 2005).

These studies focused only on the personal explanatory models of current type 2 diabetes patients. But the explanatory models of these patients were not developed in a vacuum; they were creatively constructed and are continually revised with reference to stories, metaphors, and ideas surrounding type 2 diabetes in the wider sociocultural context. This is why medical anthropologists like Kleinman expected that explanatory models would show cultural patterning. Analysis of patient explanatory models is incomplete without a portrait of this context. Yet little work has been done on the role of wider discourses on type 2 diabetes.[1] What is the inner logic of the stories Americans tell themselves about the rise of type 2 diabetes? Why do Americans think *other people* get type 2 diabetes?

Rock (2005) found that the most common framing device in North American journalistic coverage of type 2 diabetes is "*Type 2 diabetes is associated with certain groups*," and that articles associated with this framing device present "modern lifestyles as the main cause" of the diabetes crisis (Rock 2005: 1834). This section extends Rock's analysis, which focused on media portrayals, by looking to the materials patients newly diagnosed with type 2 diabetes are presented: popular guide books and the popular literature on the rise of type 2 diabetes.

Much like the news articles examined in Rock's analysis, the introductions to popular handbooks for newly diagnosed patients explain the diabetes epidemic in terms of a modernity that tempts us all with high-calorie food and the freedom to be as sedentary as we wish: "Our country, indeed the entire developed world, is facing a health epidemic of frightening proportions. It's not caused by a virus, a bacteria, or anything we can catch. Instead, this burgeoning epidemic is the result of our modern lifestyles, lives in which high-fat, sugar-filled food is everywhere we turn, in which we can go days without doing anything more strenuous than turning the key in a car or flipping channels with a remote" (Davidson & Gordon 2009: 7).

This passage, from a popular series available in grocery store checkout aisles, presents risk in universal terms. Racial, national, and socioeconomic differences in risk for type 2 diabetes are absent. The authors locate the origins of the diabetes epidemic in the availability of cheap calories and the opportunity to avoid strenuous activity, risk factors that are universal to those living in the "developed world."

The idea that modern life poses a risk to everybody is common in self-help books and pamphlets introducing the type 2 diabetes epidemic. This may take the form of labeling diabetes a global problem affecting the whole developed world, or even contrasting the low diabetes rates of populations that subsisted on "premodern" diets with skyrocketing rates once those populations were exposed to modern lifestyles and Western food (e.g., Hurley 2010; Pollan 2009; Spero 2006; Boaz 2002). The introduction to one book aimed at newly diagnosed patients and their families introduces type 2 diabetes according to this familiar frame: "Diabetes is a global health problem . . . Diabetes is concentrated where food supplies allow people to eat more calories than they need so that they develop obesity, a condition of excessive fat" (Rubin 2009: 7).

Framing diabetes as a global problem and presenting as fact the idea that it is a problem associated with *plenty* casts the epidemic as a cost of modernity borne equally by all developed nations, and all people within those nations. That this cost is borne disproportionately by lower-income, racially marginalized peoples living in economically marginalized areas of this developed nation is never mentioned in the mainstream literature aimed at patients.

If the risk for diabetes comes hand in hand with modernity and humans living in wealthy, modern societies are the ones "facing [this] health epidemic of frightening proportions," then just what is so dangerous about modern lifestyles? Popular literature on the diabetes epidemic, which has exploded in recent years, emphasizes a disharmony between the world human bodies evolved to thrive in and the modern world in which they live. In some cases, authors argue explicitly that humans are naturally suited for hunter-gatherer lifestyles. Because modern lifestyles include food surplus, sedentary work, and the stress that comes along with modern responsibilities, they are at odds with the lifestyle to which human bodies are naturally adapted.

In its more sophisticated forms, the concept of evolution is key to the premise that humans are naturally suited to hunter-gatherer lifestyles. This version is clearly articulated in *Mismatch: The Lifestyle Diseases Timebomb*, a recent work of popular science. The cover shows two stick figures, side by side. The first carries a spear. The second pushes a shopping cart. The back of the paperback edition reads: "Our evolution designed us for a world very different from that in which we live now. Within a mere instant, in evolutionary terms, we transformed our environment and created a mismatch between our world and our bodies" (Gluckman & Hanson 2006).

The thesis of *Mismatch* is a more sophisticated version of the same idea presented in the grocery store checkout aisle guide mentioned above. Where once humans had to expend energy to capture or produce food, modern lifestyles demand little more than pushing a shopping cart or, in *The Complete Idiot's Guide to Diabetes* version, "turning the key in a car." Modern, convenient lifestyles make lifestyle disease possible. Modernity kills with convenience.

Quasi-scientific language can be a powerful source of legitimacy in claims about the nature of the human body. In the United States, where the word "evolution" generates controversy, the story may be framed more softly. But while the scientific concept of evolution may be the subject of a much-decried culture war, the basic concept of adaptation to natural environments is in fact widely accepted, and is embraced by intelligent design creationists (Nakhnikian 2004). Where explicit reference to evolution is missing, there are instead oblique references to an imagined premodern past, to which human bodies were better suited: "As chronic illnesses go, diabetes is relatively new. Arthritis, in contrast, has been around forever. Cavemen had arthritis. Dinosaurs had arthritis. There was no evidence of T2D, though, prior to 10,000 years ago. It started with the rise of agriculture. Hunter-gatherers don't get diabetes, but growing grains and herding animals resulted in the consumption of more calories, more carbohydrates and more saturated fat" (Spero 2006: 10).

Rhetorical references to cavemen, the African savannah, or premodern man conjure up images of a shared natural history and further buttress the assumption that all humans in modern, resource-rich societies are at risk for type 2 diabetes. At the same time, they provide insight into the kind of lifestyle that would support a diabetes-free population.

Because the problem is that modern life does not match the lifestyle to which human bodies are best adapted, the way to stay healthy is to live in a way more similar to the life to which they *are* adapted. Portrayals of the life for which human bodies are best designed or adapted can be colorful. One of the more strident proponents of this approach claims, "Mimicking our hunter-gatherer ancestors is the best way to cure diabetes" (Boaz 2002). Less dramatically, other authors suggest lives with less stress, fewer carbohydrates, and fewer processed foods.

If the road to diabetes perdition is paved with "modern" lifestyles, the road to salvation is paved with "natural" lifestyles. In interviews, respondents also associate "natural" with health, although they are more likely to do so by expressing suspicion of processed foods than by suggesting that humans should only eat what they can manage to kill with a spear. Fast food and foods filled with chemicals rather than "real" ingredients are identified as unhealthy, while "natural," "real" foods are healthy. Asked to describe how people in America could avoid getting diabetes, a mother of two children and returning student explained, "Not so much processed food, I guess, natural, not necessarily homegrown but food that's made out of real ingredients that aren't canned, that don't have chemicals."

Participants identified "processed food" and the chemicals it contains as major barriers to leading a natural, healthy lifestyle. Importantly, the food this mother identifies as healthy does not need to be homegrown or homemade in order to qualify as natural. She is raising two children mostly on her own and has returned to school in addition to holding down a job; home cooking is out of the question most nights. Rather, "natural" is a keyword she looks for when she is buying prepared or partially prepared food for herself and her children.

The equation of "natural" with safe and "chemical" with unsafe has also long been a theme in interviews designed to draw out American patients' explanatory models (Loewe & Freeman 2000; Ferzacca 2000). With diabetes patients, this can manifest itself in the belief that medications are the proximate cause of illness. Loewe and Freeman (2000: 387) noted that some type 2 diabetes patients say in interviews that they believe that a medication administered by a biomedical professional actually precipitated their diabetes in the first place. Many health care providers interviewed for the present study noted that patient concerns about going on insulin usually stemmed from the belief that insulin had led directly to an acquaintance or relative "losing a foot" or experiencing other complications.

One endocrinology fellow I interviewed, Dr. Shaw, noted that she often must educate patients who want to lose weight but have struggled on their own and hesitate to try medication. "A lot of times people are afraid of using weight loss medications or they don't know what's in there," Dr. Shaw explained. "They don't want to use something over the counter because they're afraid it may have some crazy chemical." Dr. Shaw identified a new generation over-the-counter weight loss aid that she believes to be safe and effective, but says that she has to work hard to assure patients that it is not full of those "crazy chemicals."

This lay emphasis on the natural can be a source of great frustration for medical professionals in the United States, because some patients posit biomedicine as the opposite of natural. Nurse Waugh, a nurse practitioner with decades of experience and a mouthful of certifications, spends about twenty hours a week working with both type 1 and type 2 diabetes patients:

> NURSE WAUGH: People come in, and they want something that's natural, or they don't want it. They don't want to take a drug.
> INTERVIEWER: What does that mean, though?
> NURSE WAUGH: Okay. So they don't want to take a drug. They don't want to take any other drugs that are sort of traditional prescription drugs, but they will buy anything from some Joe Schmo in Tijuana, Mexico, as a supplement, and the supplements are not regulated. There's absolutely no guarantee of what is in there. There are people on the Internet selling hormonal extracts that are extremely dangerous to people.

Nurse Waugh is essentially observing that lay definitions of safe and biomedical definitions of safe do not always coincide. Her patients associate health and safety with the "natural" treatment, which they perceive as free of potentially harmful, unnatural chemicals because it is supposedly derived from herbs, animal extracts, or minerals. Drugs, in contrast, are seen as potentially full of these harmful, unnatural chemicals. The nurse practitioner, on the other hand, believes the drugs are safe and health-supporting based on her faith in the accurate production of safety profiles through clinical trials and their assurance by peer review. She is mystified by her patients' behavior.

But even many biomedical professionals are suspicious of the unnatural-seeming chemicals that seem to saturate modern life. For instance, when asked why the rate of type 2 diabetes seemed to be rising so rapidly in the United States, Dr. Austen, an endocrinologist, pointed to obesity as the most proximate cause. But she also theorized that the obesity epidemic could be caused not just by overeating, but also by the presence of unnatural chemicals in American fast food:

> I think it is obesity. I think obesity is increasing because we are an inside desk working culture versus an outside farming culture. I think we have access to easy food. We are a fast food culture, and I'm not sure, sometimes I almost wonder if it's not just the calories but something in that food that is intercalated with our membranes that have made us more insulin resistant, something to do with the fats that—maybe the trans-fat or just—all the fake, weird chemicals that are put in foods. (Endocrinologist)

Dr. Austen mirrored many of the same themes present in patient and popular explanations of the origins of the type 2 diabetes epidemic. She contrasts contemporary lifestyles with an imagined past and critically assesses "easy food." She is suspicious of the "fake, weird chemicals" that accompany industrial food production and processing, mirroring a popular patient theory traded on diabetes support forums that rising rates of diabetes are attributable to some sort of environmental toxin rather than dietary change.[2]

In the United States, narratives about diabetes emphasize universal risk and illustrate the perception that illness can arise when one treats the body in ways that are "unnatural," whether through a lifestyle to which the human body is poorly adapted or through the consumption of "fake, weird chemicals." Modern lifestyles thus place those who embrace them at risk of type 2 diabetes.

But all this simply means that modern individuals must work at maintaining themselves, work at resisting the temptation to succumb to a sedentary lifestyle and a life of easy processed food. In the next section, I discuss how this universal risk narrative slips so easily into a story about culpability. This section primarily explored my first question: What is the inner logic of the story Americans tell themselves about the rise of type 2 diabetes? The next addresses my second question: Why do Americans think *other people* get diabetes?

Control and Culpability: "My-Fault Diabetes"

As we sat in her sunny office in a Veterans Affairs hospital, Dr. Eliot, an endocrinologist, described her concerns about the negative assessments many type 2 diabetes patients face after their diagnosis. While she works primarily with older male African American veterans with whom she might seem to have little in common, she explained how she strives to approach them with the same sympathy and benefit of the doubt she would extend to a friend.

"I have a friend of a friend from before I was even in endocrinology, she has type 2 diabetes, and when I met her she said, 'I have my-fault diabetes,'" Dr. Eliot explained. She was taken aback that her acquaintance seemed to blame herself for a chronic disease that affected every aspect of her life. "And I'll never forget that," Dr. Eliot went on. "It made such an impression on me. And so yeah, I don't subscribe to that thinking [that places blame]."

This was the first time I had heard the term "my-fault diabetes" to differentiate type 1 diabetes from type 2 diabetes, but it would not be the last. The question of fault is itself a fault line between type 1 and type 2 patients on patient forums and support sites, where patients with the two distinct conditions sometimes mingle. Internet forums aimed at people working to manage diabetes are usually civil, supportive environments where patients exchange information, nutrition tips, and peer support.[3] When the friendly, positive tone of these forums is interrupted, it is almost always over the question of who or what is to blame for type 2 diabetes. These fault discussions run hundreds of posts long and, in sharp contrast to the positive overall tone of the support forums, are emotional and even acrimonious.[4] When the question of fault emerges, type 1 diabetes patients argue that "the science" shows that lifestyle factors lead to type 2 diabetes, while type 2 diabetes patients accuse the type 1 diabetes patients of self-righteousness and a sense of moral superiority.

Providers, consciously or unconsciously, may contribute to the moral divide between type 1 and type 2 diabetes. Anecdotes about the subtle and not-so-subtle ways that providers rank their patients with metabolic and renal disorders abound. One physician, intending to comfort the family of a woman on dialysis when her kidneys failed following a massive infection, told her son that everyone at the dialysis center was sympathetic because, unlike most of the dialysis patients, her renal failure "wasn't her fault." Posters to support forums share occasional stories about harsh, judgmental health care providers.[5]

In interviews, providers said that this sort of explicit moralizing is probably rare, but candidly pointed out that it is difficult not to sympathize more with type 1 diabetes patients, who played no role in producing their condition, than with type 2 patients, whom they view as having played some (if limited) role in producing their condition. Dr. Hardy, an endocrinology fellow, reflected that while it was exceedingly rare for his colleagues at a university medical center to explicitly use moral language to differentiate between patients with type 1 and type 2 diabetes, it was hard not to recognize a difference in the etiology of the two conditions.

> Just to give you an example, maybe late-onset type 1 diabetes where
> it's an autoimmune diabetes. It's nothing they did to bring it on, versus
> a patient who is extremely obese and has never followed a particular
> diet or taken any medication. And not to say you look at one or the
> other with more sympathy exactly, but . . . There's definitely with
> diabetes a particular . . . A lot of it is sort of self-inflicted, so, of
> course, you kind of think about that a little differently. (Endocrinology
> fellow)

Dr. Hardy, whom colleagues repeatedly identified in interviews as an example of a doctor who is particularly gifted at communicating with patients, suggested that most of the difference between provider approaches to type 1 and type 2 diabetes patients is subtle and perhaps even unconscious. In other parts of his interview, he emphasized that a good doctor is someone who does well by his patients regardless of how he evaluates them personally.

American health professionals carefully distinguish their type 1 patients from type 2 patients, not only in disease etiology but also by personality type. Dr. Austen, an elegant endocrinologist at a university medical center, reflected that even though she routinely explained the etiology of type 2 diabetes as primarily genetic, she sometimes catches herself thinking or saying small things that suggest that these patients are guilty of some moral failure. This narrative is so pervasive in popular culture that she must police herself to make sure it doesn't affect her patient care. Sitting in her office one afternoon, she said she could even think of a point earlier that same day where she caught herself making that assumption.

"Today we were just talking about the [high] no-show rate of someone's clinic, and she's got mostly type 2s. I said, 'That's how they got that diabetes.'" She paused before going on. "Probably it's genetics . . . Sometimes you'll have the same body weight person, same sedentary lifestyle and you have the wrong genes and the other person doesn't . . ." She trailed off.

Dr. Austen is torn between two stories about why these patients developed type 2 diabetes while others did not. Her first, unprocessed reaction is that the same laziness or relaxed attitude that she believes led them to skip appointments put them at higher risk for their disease. But she catches herself and qualifies her explanation with a genetic narrative. Still, after this qualification she returns a second time to the issue of the patients' personality:

> With [my colleague's] clinic, I just said, "They have the type B personality." They just forget or like they—they got busy, didn't want to really cancel, and so she had five people . . . The first five people didn't show in her clinic. It's kind of a personality. (Endocrinologist)

As an experienced medical researcher in addition to her practice, Dr. Austen was careful to point out that the etiology of type 2 diabetes in a given patient is complicated, and that while lifestyle factors such as overeating and too little physical activity directly affect the chances that a person will develop diabetes, the relationship between patient behavior and diabetes is mediated by genetic risk. Still, she continually returned to the issue of personality, associating type 2 diabetes patients with a lack of initiative or discipline.

Lay narratives about the origins of type 2 diabetes are also linked to underlying discourses about morality and the self. Clearly, the ethic of individual responsibility and discipline runs throughout American discourses on the growth of type 2 diabetes. Rock (2005) found in a qualitative analysis of two American magazines and two Canadian newspapers that the most common framing device in journalistic coverage of type 2 diabetes is *"Type 2 diabetes is associated with certain groups."* The articles associated with this framing device present "modern lifestyles as the main cause" and "stressed informed individual choice" as a remedy (Rock 2005: 1834).

In lay interviews, sympathy for people with diabetes one knows personally was mixed with a sense that patients bear responsibility not only for having developed diabetes, but also for failing to manage their condition so as not to develop complications. Jackie, a 30-year-old parole officer in rural North Carolina, described her reaction when a colleague had to retire after losing his foot to complications of type 2 diabetes:

> He wasn't taking his medication and he was eating candy. I love [colleague] to death, but he was an idiot. It's that thing where I can't help you if you can't help yourself. (Parole officer)

Earlier and later in her interview, Jackie blamed corporations, chemicals, and marketing for both the epidemic of obesity and the growth of type 2 diabetes in the United States. When asked if she blamed anyone or anything for the unhealthy lifestyle she said she saw all around her, she answered laughingly, "What's the name of the guy who invented marketing?" But her evaluation of her colleague with diabetes is more complex. While Jackie may be angry at McDonald's and corporate America for enabling Americans to eat huge portions of what she called processed, unnatural food, she also reserved some harsh words for the person she knows living with type 2 diabetes. Her colleague, she said, is an "idiot" for allowing himself to become so ill and for persisting in eating candy and ignoring the medication his doctors recommended. There is plenty of fault to go around.

In *Illness as Metaphor*, Susan Sontag notes that illnesses have always been ranked by the degree to which the people they affect are perceived to be morally responsible for their own suffering (Sontag 1978, cited in Broom & Whittaker 2004). The difference between evaluations of those living with type

1 and type 2 diabetes dramatically demonstrates the role of moral responsibility in these assessments.

If the origins of the type 2 diabetes epidemic are located explicitly in the availability of cheap calories and the opportunity to avoid strenuous activity, then they are also implicitly located in the choice of some people to indulge in those cheap calories and avoidance of activity. If stress and the temptations of comfort food and a sedentary lifestyle are universal risks to modern humans in technologically advanced countries, then there must be some explanation for why some fall to temptation and others do not. After all, a third of Americans may be obese — but that means that two-thirds are not obese. Those who fall to so-called lifestyle diseases are thus imagined to be in some way responsible for their disease.

Obesity plays a major role in coloring the moral narrative about type 2 diabetes. News segments, books, informational pamphlets, and respondents repeatedly link the diabetes epidemic to obesity. Diabetes patients have been shown to internalize this, incorporating obesity linked to overindulgence or failure of discipline in their explanatory models. One interviewee cited in Broom and Whittaker (2004: 2374) told researchers, "I think diabetes is just fat people eating too much fat." The rhetorical linking of obesity, lack of self-control, and illness makes it all too easy to cast the type 2 diabetes epidemic as a morality tale about personal responsibility, at great cost to patients living with the disease.

Of Race and Risk

One difficulty with the very idea of a wider narrative on the origins of the type 2 diabetes epidemic in the United States is that the United States is an extraordinarily diverse country and the type 2 diabetes epidemic is anything but evenly distributed across it. African Americans are nearly 1.8 times more likely than Caucasians to suffer from type 2 diabetes (American Diabetes Association 2011). The CDC estimates that an astonishing 18.7 percent of non-Hispanic African Americans over the age of twenty live with diabetes (National Diabetes Factsheet 2011). In comparison, 10.2 percent of non-Hispanic Caucasian Americans are thought to be living with the disease.

Diabetes education materials produced for and by African Americans present a slightly different narrative about the origins of the epidemic, not only because African Americans are statistically at greater risk for the disease but also because reflections on the natural history of humanity so frequently conjure up images of the African savannah. While Caucasian Americans use such images to emphasize the universality of risk and shared heritage as humans, African American materials use the same images to demonstrate the social context of diabetes risk.

The Black Health Library Guide to Diabetes, for example, uses images of African hunter-gatherers leading an ancient lifestyle as the prototype for a diabetes-free lifestyle: "Across the sunbaked sands of the Sahara desert travel a race of people whose day-to-day lives, like those of their ancestors, are relatively untouched by Western influences. They are the Broayas, a small but unique tribe of nomads. Dark-skinned and straight-haired, they are blessed with extraordinary physical endurance and no obesity. They also have no diabetes" (Henry & Johnson 1993: 31).

This story is almost identical to the one portrayed in mainstream diabetes guides. But the purpose of this rhetorical image is not to reaffirm the universality of risk for diabetes for all modern humans because of a shared natural history. Rather, the explicit purpose of the anecdote about Africans who have hung on to their premodern way of life is to illustrate that African Americans are not constitutionally vulnerable to type 2 diabetes. As the book goes on to argue, "For some races, the evidence that diabetes runs along racial lines is undeniable. But that's not the case for African-Americans. If it were, black Africans would have the same high rates of diabetes that African-Americans have. In reality, Africans have relatively little diabetes" (Henry & Johnson 1993: 32).

The argument, then, is that type 2 diabetes is not really a racial disease in the sense of genetic risk, though African Americans' high rates of the disease may at first make it appear that way. Social structure—not biological structure—renders African Americans at higher risk than other Americans. This stands in contrast to the narrative presented in materials produced for nonspecific American audiences, where the epidemic is framed as a cost of modernity, a risk borne equally by all developed nations and all people within those nations. The recognition that this cost is borne disproportionately by marginalized peoples is specific to literature aimed at the specialized audience of African American diabetes patients.

The language of choice is also different in this version of the diabetes epidemic's story. It is the lifestyle that African Americans have been *subjected* to that explains the higher risk for type 2 diabetes in the African American community. "And so for our grandparents' parents, the act of being forcibly uprooted and thrust in the midst of a new culture, with new foods, and new labor-saving machines, may have set the stage for a present-day diabetes epidemic that began to appear as black folks adopted more western ways" (Henry & Johnson 1993: 33).

It is not that choice plays no role in this narrative. However, choice is situated within a broader (and, at least initially, foreign) social context that powerfully shapes the lifestyle factors contributing to African Americans' higher risk for illness. As we will see in the next chapter, this narrative is much closer to Japanese explanations of the type 2 diabetes epidemic than the narratives that dominate other American health materials.

Conclusions

The most common American narrative about the origins of the diabetes epidemic emphasizes the universality of diabetes risk to all people living modern lifestyles. This narrative suggests that illness arises when one treats the body in ways that are unnatural, such as by consuming heavily processed foods full of chemicals, overeating, or not having to work for one's food as ancestral hunter-gatherers did. Paradoxically, because risk is treated as universal to those who must live modern lifestyles, those that fall to so-called lifestyle diseases may be imagined to be in some way personally responsible for their disease. All who live modern lifestyles are at greater risk for diabetes but only some succumb. Further, diabetes is frequently related to obesity, with moral overtones that overshadow the socioeconomic and genetic patterning of diabetes risk. In contrast, patient literature produced by and for African Americans provides a powerful alternative narrative that emphasizes that risk is not borne equally by those living in contemporary America.

Few scholars have addressed lay narratives about the origin of diabetes as expressed by those who do not have a current diabetes diagnosis, and little work has been done on the discourse surrounding diabetes that patients encounter when they first receive a diagnosis themselves. The stories patients encounter about the origins of diabetes in the population — rather than in their own personal experience — can significantly affect the ways in which patients themselves frame explanations of the disease's appearance in their own lives. This chapter attempted to provide some of that necessary context.

The explanation of diabetes risk as universal to all people living under modern circumstances, the language about modern man's ill adaptation to modern convenience, and the implication of personal lifestyle "choices" in the elevated diabetes risk of certain groups may seem unremarkable, even familiar. It is a story that makes intuitive *sense* to many Americans, whether the journalists in Rock's (2005) study, or the doctors, laypeople, and producers and consumers of the diabetes literature discussed here. This narrative represents largely unexamined beliefs and assumptions—easy answers—proffered by people who have not lived with diabetes themselves. Easy answers are easy because they are at the top of the cultural tool kit. The next chapter, however, shows that Japanese respondents and popular literature offer a very different story about the origins and nature of the diabetes epidemic.

CHAPTER THREE

Our Genes Don't Match Your Culture
Japanese Narratives about the Origins of Type 2 Diabetes

Theories of medicalization and biomedicalization have generated new perspectives on the processes transforming biomedicine and expanding its domain beyond illness to health itself. Although most empirical work engaging with the biomedicalization framework is still U.S.-based, biomedicalization scholars have always argued that medicalization and biomedicalization are not merely North American phenomena. Rather, "these transformations of medical care and of life itself are, of course, increasingly exported and (re)modeled as well as being produced elsewhere . . ." (Clarke et al. 2010: 32). This chapter examines medicalization and biomedicalization in their "transnational travels" by analyzing the construction of the type 2 diabetes epidemic in contemporary Japan. I use grounded theory to situate and model the ways in which risk for diabetes is explained by Japanese health professionals, patients, and other lay participants during interviews. In the process, I draw connections between differences in the biomedicalized production of risk for diabetes in Japan and broader social patterns that provide the raw material from which risk is conceived and constructed.

Like the United States, Japan is among the world's most affluent societies, and the dominant approach to health care and maintenance is technologically advanced biomedicine. The Japanese and American medical communities share similar empirical, often reductionist, approaches to the production and adjudication of best practices in medicine. And decades of exchange programs, fellowships, and cooperation agreements between Japanese and American universities have brought generations of Japanese physicians to American medical centers on a temporary basis.

However, these similarities have limits. As Shobita Parthasarathy (2012) demonstrates in her work on BRCA testing in Britain and the United States, we should not assume that shared emphasis on empirical medicine will necessarily lead to identical conclusions about best practices; the influence of national context on practice can be profound. As an example of technoscientific biomedicine outside the West, Japan has much to contribute to North American scholars' expanding understanding of biomedicalization.

As I argued in Chapter 1, biomedicalization has progressed in Japan along several of the dimensions articulated by others (see Clarke et al. 2003, 2010). The focus on health has intensified, and states of pre-illness or potential illness have been demarcated, denormalized, and increasingly managed through biomedical intervention. This is particularly true of diabetes: in Japan, it is common for patients to be diagnosed and managed for impaired glucose tolerance (IGT) years before they develop type 2 diabetes. Second, the intensifying emphasis on surveillance and risk, particularly for age-related changes, puts Japan at the forefront of global biomedicalization. Most laypeople are able to articulate surprisingly detailed risk profiles for chronic disease and turn to biomedicine not only to diagnose and treat these diseases, but as the authoritative source for insight into the lifestyle that will prevent them and maintain normality. Finally, the production of risk is a key feature of biomedicalization in both the United States and Japan, yet it is constituted differently in the two countries. As a consequence, the implied moral imperative to manage that risk is also constructed differently—shaping how people with diabetes are assessed by their health care providers and peers.

The public health narrative casting the increase in type 2 diabetes and IGT as an epidemic—and an epidemic with a clear source—is part of this production of risk. The interviews analyzed in this chapter document the construction of the type 2 diabetes "epidemic" by laypeople, diabetes patients, and biomedical health professionals. Interview participants cast Japan's diabetes epidemic as a morality tale about the nature of Japanese identity, mirroring a trope that stretches back at least as far as Japan's modernization period. In stark contrast to the American diabetes epidemic narrative explicated in the previous chapter, this narrative emphasizes the particularity of diabetes risk to the Japanese body in contemporary, globalized Japan.

In the following sections, interview respondents respond to questions about how diabetes came to be an epidemic in Japan. Many use culture as an explanatory device. The idea that Japanese culture is essentially unique has long been rejected by most social scientists and theorists. However, this theme is pervasive in popular discourse. Explanation and belief are not the same thing. The fact that a narrative is pervasive does not mean it is in earnest. Pervasiveness is important, though, because it indicates the explanation that is easiest or closest at hand.

Lay participants described the Japanese body as uniquely, evolutionarily adapted to traditional Japanese food and lifestyle practices, and thus maladapted to "foreign" elements such as meat and oil. They argue, in effect, that the Japanese body is uniquely hyperadapted to Japanese food culture and vice versa, and that the body becomes imbalanced and polluted by foods and practices that are not historically Japanese. Importantly, these respondents described non-Japanese foods as suitable for non-Japanese bodies but as unsuitable for Japanese bodies. Physicians and other providers participate in and reinforce this explanatory mechanism by emphasizing an evolutionary explanation for high diabetes risk in interactions with patients, mixing evolutionary fables that emphasize shared Japanese identity with technoscientific references to genetic risk.

The claims of Japanese cultural and physiological uniqueness that surface in conversations about the diabetes epidemic — and the evolutionary fables that lend them authority — reference a long-popular discourse in Japan. In the next section, I briefly outline the discourse on Japanese uniqueness (typically referred to as *nihonjinron*) and engage some contemporary analyses of it. The purpose of this foray is to introduce the reader to the trope that many interview respondents reference, rendering their explanations more legible. I then turn to the interviews, analyzing the most frequent explanations of diabetes risk in light of popular *nihonjinron* discourse. Finally, I examine the ways in which lay and biomedical professional narratives about the origins of the diabetes epidemic reinforce one another, the popular sense that Japanese physiology and culture are uniquely intertwined, and a shared understanding of risk that is both biomedicalized and rooted in a local cultural tool kit.

Nihonjinron: How the Japanese Talk about Being Japanese

Nihonjinron refers broadly to the body of popular and intellectual literature that explicates and examines the origins of the Japanese people's purported uniqueness. Japan's thriving publishing industry produces and markets new popular books on topics that are supposedly uniquely Japanese each year, from neurologists claiming that Japanese social practices shape their brains (Hayashi 2009) to ruminations on the effect of Japan's four seasons on Japanese society's approach to death and dying. *Nihonjinron* produced by Japanese authors has variously asserted that because Japan is an island nation, its people have evolved as a distinct race (Watanabe 1954; Dale 2012), that the Japanese language is a linguistic isolate that conditions native speakers to think in uniquely Japanese ways that no foreigner, no matter how fluent, can understand (Tsukimoto 2008), and that the Japanese form relationships of dependence that reject boundaries between the self and others (Doi 1981; Dale 1986). *Nihonjinron* cultural products make commonplace the idea that

Japanese are profoundly *different* from the rest of the world, not only cultur-ally but physiologically.[1] Regardless of whether or not they believe it, these ideas are familiar to most adults in Japan.

Some scholars have argued that the historical context of the birth of *ni-honjinron* discourse during Japan's modernization period facilitated a fusion of racialized and cultural determinisms that persists today. Yoshino (2005) argued that in the prewar period "ideas of culture developed alongside im-passioned debates about racial boundaries and racial origins. These in turn helped to refine and popularize a sense of the Japanese as a distinct 'ethnic group'—*minzoku*—a concept which fused images of race with images of cul-ture." Japan's particular heritage as a racially othered imperial power along-side the club of European colonial powers in the early decades of the twentieth century may have contributed to the popular sense that the Japanese were profoundly different from other nations.

Of particular concern to *nihonjinron* producers and consumers during Ja-pan's colonial period was the relationship between Japan and the West on the one hand, and Japan and the rest of Asia on the other. A racial outsider to the industrialized nations of other continents but a colonial power in its own region, this dual position was a continual site of conflict for Japan, cul-turally as well as politically. *Nihonjinron* discourse is historically concerned with establishing Japan's place in the world in relation to Asia; it character-izes, displaces, and continually rearticulates Japan as "in but above" and "sim-ilar but superior to" Asia (Iwabuchi 2002). Distinguishing Japanese from other Asians, racially as well as culturally, and positioning them as the right-ful leaders of Asia and equals of Western powers, was a major discursive project of modernizing Japan (Yoshino 1992; Iwabuchi 2002). Arguments about the nature of "Japanese-ness" were a vehicle for intellectuals and every-day Japanese subjects to explore the contours, causes, and consequences of Japan's unique position in the colonial world.

Some Japan scholars have argued that this historical context contributed to a fusion of the cultural and the physiological that persists today—a ten-dency to conflate cultural and physiological traits (Dale 2012; Morris-Suzuki 1998; McVeigh 2004). Even in contemporary *nihonjinron*, culture is often imagined to be embodied in Japanese physiology, as in the argument that the Japanese language is associated with unique brain function (see Tsunoda 1978; Dale 1986). In other words, *nihonjinron* cosmology can suggest that cul-tural Japanese-ness begot physiological Japanese-ness: Japanese culture forms Japanese bodies.

But most Japan scholars have focused on the more common claim in discourse on uniqueness: the claim that the physical environment has simultaneously influenced both the physicality of the Japanese and Japanese culture itself (Dale 2012). The Japanese environment is said to have shaped Japanese physiology, resulting in a small-statured race habituated to eating fish, as well as to have shaped Japanese culture, resulting, for instance, in a culture with a supposedly unique appreciation of nature, the ephemeral, and the subtle. Descriptions of supposed physiological and cultural uniqueness in *nihonjinron* writings often locate the origin of difference in a particular Japanese experience of nature (Morris-Suzuki 1998; McVeigh 2004).

The Japanese body, culture, and nation are inextricably linked in much popular and intellectual discourse in Japan. This conceptual fusion persists well beyond the shelves of *kokugaku* sections of bookstores. It is imagined that any person who meets one criterion will naturally meet the others. In this cosmology, Japanese nationality presupposes Japanese physiology and culture; this can be observed in Japan's blood-based approach to citizenship (Ortloff & Frey 2007) and insistence that families that have lived in Japan for generations with Korean names give them up for proper Japanese ones before receiving citizenship (Nahm 1988; Min 1992). And Japanese physiology presupposes Japanese culture and nation, as is suggested by Japan's preferential acceptance (driven by economic necessity) of economic migrants who could prove a Japanese bloodline because, it was argued, they would "fit in" (Tsuda 2003). In this discourse, the Japanese nation, Japanese bodies, and Japanese culture are imagined to overlap sufficiently that if someone is identified as Japanese in one sense they can naturally be assumed to be Japanese in the others as well.

Given the ubiquity of this discourse, it is easy for some in Japan to assume that Japanese identity is a single package, in which nation, body, and culture are coterminous. Nation, body, and culture may be recognized to be discrete categories in the abstract but are not in practice. Individuals and groups who do not reflect this trinity—and there are many—become profoundly unsettling. Brazilian-Japanese guest workers, Japanese nationals raised overseas, children of mixed parentage, and Japan's Korean minority all upset the correspondence among these categories. The interruption of the ontological fusion between nation, body, and culture makes these groups objects of popular interest and moral uncertainty.[2] When Japanese nationality, physiology, and home culture do not line up, the result is expected to be dysfunction.

The interruption of this ontological fusion of nation, body, and culture is referenced in much discourse on diabetes risk in Japan. Saying is not believing. But saying still matters. As biomedical professionals and laypeople frame the diabetes epidemic, many approach it through a preexisting model that is within easy reach: *nihonjinron*-inflected stories about the nature of Japanese bodies that pervade popular culture. In these just-so stories, Japanese bodies are not only unique from foreign bodies but also inextricably tied to and dependent on Japanese culture and nation. This model posits that when the three, mutually dependent elements of Japanese identity are thrown into disharmony, the result is a failure to thrive — illness.

Because this narrative is so pervasive, it is easy for respondents to explain diabetes as a consequence of growing disharmony between two of the three elements of that trinity: the Japanese body and Japanese culture. As above, saying is not believing. But saying still matters. To associate managing and maintaining health with being a good Japanese, even as a matter of explanatory convenience, adds further weight to the moral imperative to maintain a state of health. Interview participants and other informants describe the Japanese body as uniquely, evolutionarily adapted to traditional Japanese food and lifestyle practices, and thus maladapted to certain "foreign" elements such as meat, oil, and bread. Respondents suggest, in effect, that the Japanese body, adapted to Japanese food culture, becomes imbalanced and polluted by foods and practices that are not Japanese. When the Japanese body is no longer aligned with Japanese culture, its fate becomes uncertain.

Health care providers reference and reinforce this explanatory model when they emphasize an evolutionary explanation for high diabetes risk in the Japanese population. Because the Japanese body is adapted to a diet of fish and rice, they explain, it is at a higher risk for diabetes in the context of a westernizing food culture that contains foreign elements such as meat and oil. Japanese foods thought to contribute to diabetes risk in U.S. circles, such as white rice and bento-style convenience fare, are erased from this discourse. Biomedical professionals and educators thus employ a standard, globally recognized evolutionary explanation for risk in a way that has distinct local meanings.

Body and Culture in Disharmony

The interviews suggest that a narrative about disharmony between Japanese bodies and the encroachment of foreign cultural influences is the most common approach to explaining the diabetes epidemic in Japan. This narrative curates elements of *nihonjinron* discourse on Japanese identity but is couched in the logic of evolution and the technoscientific language of blood glucose, pancreatic function, and genotype. Even as the processes of biomedicalization shape the ways in which diabetes is constructed and talked about, the contexts of Japanese identity politics and attendant assumptions about the origins of dysfunction shape many of the underlying assumptions and values that biomedicalization reinforces.

In the interviews, respondents were asked to discuss their personal ideas about the origins of type 2 diabetes in Japan and around the world, impressions of people with diabetes, beliefs about prevention, and opinions regarding the effectiveness of various treatment options. Many respondents hypothesized that the prehistoric Japanese physical environment is the source of a unique Japanese cultural and physiological heritage, and that Japanese culture maintains uniquely Japanese bodies. Medical as well as lay interviewees' emphasis on the particularity of diabetes risk to Japanese bodies was sharply different from discussions of risk in American popular discourse and interviews. Japanese interviewees perceived diabetes risk as something faced particularly by Japanese as a people. While American respondents referred generally to "people" or "humans" when discussing risk, Japanese respondents referred to "the Japanese." And while American respondents frequently cited disharmony between human bodies and modernity to explain illness and strategies for health maintenance, Japanese respondents typically referenced disharmony between *Japanese* bodies and a culture they saw as increasingly incorporating foreign influences.

In the following section, I present and analyze the most common lay narratives about the origins of diabetes in the Japanese interview set. These narratives reference a disconnect between Japanese bodies and Japanese food culture as a source of illness. Next, I discuss the narratives embedded in explanations of the origins of diabetes presented by physicians, nurses, and co-medicals such as nutritionists, and examine the ways in which these narratives rely on and reify the model shared by most lay respondents. The responses evidence intensive biomedicalization—through the recourse to technoscientific modes of measurement and language, the emphasis on states of risk, and the (re)production of knowledge in part through the interaction of technoscience and preoccupation with risk. However, the underlying moral narrative about the origins of the epidemic is different from the predominant U.S. narrative about type 2 diabetes, inflected with different assumptions and the marks of different cultural tool kits.

Lay Narratives

When asked why rates of diabetes were rising in Japan, lay respondents often posit that their bodies are evolved to a Japanese cultural milieu that is rapidly being lost (or has already been lost) to westernization. Explanations of the origins of the diabetes epidemic repeatedly return to three key themes. First, they employ popular notions of evolution to explain why the Japanese body and Japanese food naturally go together. Second, they identify Western-style food as the most proximate cause for diabetes in Japan, rather than changing patterns in the consumption of Japanese-style food. Finally, they distinguish Western bodies from Japanese bodies, positing that Western foods are suitable for Western bodies but not for Japanese bodies. As I note above, the easy explanation may not be a deeply held belief, but it nonetheless has consequences for everyday practice.

Co-evolution of the Japanese Body and Japanese Culture

As in the United States, respondents drew on popularized concepts of biological evolution. Junichi, a successful businessman and owner of an elder-care facility in his midseventies, explained:

> Japanese people's origins in primeval times, at a time when people were close to monkeys . . . At that time, the lifestyle of Japan's people was to eat seeds, fruits, and roots—things like that. [Those were our] ancestors, and we have their constitution. In the West, people have inherited the constitution of their ancestors who ate meat from long, long ago, right?[3] (Businessman and owner of retirement home, rural Japan)

Junichi collapsed prehistorical time, tracing Japan's origins all the way to a time when "people were close to monkeys." His phrasing mirrored arguments about Japan's purported racial purity made by conservative commentators like Shoichi Watanabe, even though Junichi himself was neither a nationalist or nor culturally conservative. While Junichi abhorred nationalist politics and carefully referred to distant ancestors as "Japan's people" rather than "Japanese," the idea that Japanese people evolved to a *distinct* diet on the Japanese archipelago for as long as humans could be considered human struck him as natural, unproblematic, and scientific.

For most respondents, evolution explained why Japanese bodies are specifically suited to Japanese food. Yui, a thirty-eight-year-old upper-middle-class mother who spent several years of her childhood abroad while her father ran his company's Southeast Asian operations, explained:

> As for being prone to diabetes, it's probably that Japanese people ate Japanese things—fish, miso soup, vegetables. So Japanese people's bodies were formed to match those foods. However, since a different culture has become mainstream, the body and the food it consumes no longer suit one another. They don't match, and so there is diabetes.[4] (Volunteer translator and stay-at-home mother, urban Japan)

Yui referenced the idea that the physical reality and cultural heritage of premodern Japan worked together seamlessly to produce the Japanese. Seamlessly, the story goes, until modernization with its Western trappings brought foreign foods and new lifestyles to Japan. Then the Japanese body—previously in such harmony with the Japanese lifestyle—was shifted out of balance.

The problem is not the Japanese genetic heritage; rather, the problem is the disharmony between that heritage and contemporary Japan. An urban man in his thirties explained in English:

> We used to [be healthy] because we have very good genes. But it turned out we don't have genes against those—all the caloried food . . . We are genetically very bad against nowadays' food. We are less competitive that way. (Urban professional)

This respondent made a claim common in interviews: that Japanese genes are essentially "good," but they are ill-adapted to contemporary diet. His explanation highlights the flipside of the idea that Japanese are uniquely hyperadapted—that the very traits and features that can be seen as evidence of Japanese uniqueness or superiority are caught in delicate balance with their context. According to its logic, the very traits that evidence Japanese racial-cultural superiority in one context can handicap in others.

Many respondents mentioned the idea that Japanese bodies are physiologically unique as a result of evolution. Very occasionally, respondents drew explicitly on *nihonjinron* articles of faith, such as the retired businessman and his wife who hypothesized that Japanese were at higher risk for diabetes when they ate "rich" Western food because Japanese intestines are of a different length than those of foreigners. Japanese intestines, they argued, are longer than foreigners' intestines because the Japanese historically ate a vegetarian diet. They explained that long intestines are well adapted for a diet of vegetables high in fiber but not for "American steaks." The "Japanese intestines are longer than foreign intestines" idea is familiar to consumers of popular *nihonjinron*. While the claim is less usual in literature on diabetes, it has long been a staple of television quiz shows and medical documentaries in Japan. Tsutomu Hata made the claim internationally famous in 1987, when in his capacity as a former agriculture minister he told Washington that Japan could not accept imported American beef because Japanese have uniquely long intestines, rendering the consumption of too much beef dangerous (Haberman 1988). Hata later became the eightieth prime minister of Japan.

More commonly, lay respondents mirrored *nihonjinron* structures and assumptions without explicitly marshaling classic *nihonjinron* arguments, to which few subscribed. While most interviewees aligned Japanese food and food culture with Japanese bodies, they did not explicitly reference *nihonjinron* texts or thinkers. Instead, they cited their own vague impressions (*insho*) and feelings (*kanjiru*). Like Junichi and Yui, quoted above, respondents did not see themselves as consumers and certainly not as proponents of *nihonjinron* arguments. Still, they mirrored the symbolic structure of these arguments when they talked about the origins of type 2 diabetes. *Nihonjinron*-based ideas about the Japanese body are part of respondents' cultural tool kits, drawn out when they are useful for making sense of the problem at hand, not self-conscious or closely held ideologies.

Japanese Bodies and Western Food

It should already be apparent that the pervasive popular explanation for the diabetes epidemic is not only that the Japanese body is prone to diabetes but that the Japanese body is prone to diabetes in the context of a nontraditional food culture. According to this model, Japanese bodies, having been formed according to an ancient Japanese food culture, face the risk of falling to illness when they stray too far:

> Ah, yes, of course, thousands of years ago—tens of thousands of years ago—Japanese people developed their dietary lifestyle (*shokuseikatsu*) and their bodies were formed according to it. I think that an excess of sugar or fat . . . consume that sort of thing and the body is prone to [diabetes]. I wonder . . . Actually, I feel like that's the sort of thing I've heard about [its origins].[5] (Graduate student, urban Japan)

> We're Japanese people, so shouldn't we return to our original Japanese food lifestyle? Of course, Japanese food isn't the best, but for

Japanese people Japanese food is just a little more . . . [trails off][6] (Restaurant owner, rural Japan)

Respondents identified the same nutritional culprits as American interviewees—sugar and fat—but they framed them in different ways by repeatedly referencing what they imagined to be a vanishing historical food culture shared by the Japanese as a people. A plurality of respondents (47 percent), lay and medical professional alike, including both quoted above, use the word *shokuseikatsu* (literally "food lifestyle") to refer to ancient diet rather than *shokuji* (food), *tabemono* (food), or *nichijo no inshokubutsu* (daily dietary intake). *Shokuseikatsu* carries connotations of culture; it is closer in meaning to "eating habits" or "lifestyle" than to diet in a nutritional sense. *Shokuseikatsu* invokes both the nutritional and cultural content of food.

Further, sugar and fat are not merely threats to the Japanese body—they are *foreign* threats to the Japanese body. Overwhelmingly, respondents identified Western food as the most proximate explanation for rising diabetes rates. When asked why the rate of diabetes is rising in Japan, a woman who was diagnosed with diabetes in her midfifties responded:

Western food, of course. The westernization of food. From their origins, Japanese people had Japanese food.[7] (Small business owner, urban Japan)

There is certainly a good argument to be made that the westernization of the Japanese diet has contributed to rising diabetes rates; it is frequently repeated in the pages of public health journals. Diabetes educators and specialists are quick to point out that the proportion of calories coming from fat climbed steeply in the postwar era, though total caloric intake has remained relatively stable. The American occupation, economic globalization, and the prosperity that followed connected Japan to an increasingly global fast food culture. The lay respondent quoted above, like many physicians and public health experts, located the beginning of the shift toward Western food in the early part of the Showa period—the same period when the proportion of calories from fat began to rise.

But the reality is not so simple, especially since when most respondents were pressed to specify the meaning of "westernization" they referred to conspicuously foreign *styles* of food such as hamburgers and pasta rather than changing portion sizes. The average store-bought, Japanese-style bento lunchbox in Japan contains anywhere from 500 to a whopping 1,335 calories,[8] for example, while a hamburger at a Japanese McDonald's clocks in at 275 calories[9] and a quarter-pounder with cheese clocks in at 556 calories.[10] Bento boxes, ramen stands, *tonkatsu* joints, and *donburi* chains like Yoshinoya serve up some of the most meat-, carbohydrate-, and calorie-packed convenience food available.[11] Yet it is foreign styles of food that are identified as high in calories due to sugar and fat. The perception gap between calories in Japanese fast foods and Western fast foods is so great that McDonald's Japan produces tray liners detailing the calories in several of its most popular products side-by-side with traditional convenience foods. The McDonald's products invariably have fewer calories.

The rest of the fast food industry has encouraged the perception that Western food is harmful to the body while Asian food is healthy or even healing. Ajisen Ramen, a national chain, markets itself in Japan with the catch-phrase "Making food that is not only delicious, but good for you."[12] Ajisen markets itself on the basis of the supposed healing properties of its ingredients through 医食同源 (*ishokudogen*), an ancient Chinese approach to healing and preventing illness by eating "balanced" and "delicious" food. In this context, "balanced" refers to the balance of ingredients and tastes according to correspondences set out in traditional Chinese medical philosophy (Mayanagi 1998). In any other context, "balanced" would be a misnomer when applied to Ajisen dishes. While Ajisen does not publish the nutritional content of its products, chains serving similar *tonkatsu* broth ramen dishes do; similar lunch bowls at Tenkaippin Ramen, which also advertises its dishes as healthy, contain between 800 and 1,100 calories each.[13]

Ethnographic studies of fast food culture in Japan have found that Japanese participants frequently equate fast food with Western-style food but not with more traditional Japanese convenience foods (Traphagan & Brown 2002). Thus hamburgers and pizza are unquestionably fast food, but ramen, bento boxes, and sushi occupy more ambiguous territory (Traphagan & Brown 2002: 122). In interviews, several respondents mused that one of the reasons for the ubiquity of Western food in Japan is simply that Western food is convenient, whereas Japanese food takes time and "must be prepared by hand." One rural respondent in her seventies, for example, associated westernization with convenience food and Japanese food with "slow" food. "In a word, it's westernization, isn't it?" she asked rhetorically. "Yes. So now what I'm talking about is slow food—I want to return people to Japanese food . . ."[14] Western food and industrially processed foods are frequently conflated here: Japanese food is homemade by definition, while Western food is convenience food.

Once patients are labeled prediabetic or are instructed by their doctor to exercise more caution with regard to their daily caloric intake, most quickly reach the conclusion that even Japanese convenience food is not very good for them. But it is important that people who have not yet had any reason to closely monitor caloric content have the impression that Western food and Japanese food exist at opposite ends of a spectrum, where Western food is dangerous and Japanese food healthy. Vague but widespread impressions of what is healthy and what is not shape daily practices for the majority of the population. They also suggest that, all other things being equal, the more proximate a product or practice is to conceptions of Japanese culture, the more healthy—and, thus, morally good—it is assumed to be.

Western Food for Western Bodies

While respondents connected high risk for type 2 diabetes in Japan with straying from traditional diet, Westerners were thought to largely escape risk for similar reasons. Several assumed that Western bodies were evolutionarily suited to this risky diet.

> In the past . . . Oh, how to put it? Instead of meat, Japanese people ate things like rice and vegetables. So the calories were low. And then the liver . . . the liver or the pancreas making insulin? [With that diet] even when the functional capability [of the liver and pancreas] diminished, it was fine. However, today's dietary lifestyle is nothing but meat and high-calorie foods. I think that people like Americans and Westerners, they've eaten that sort of diet forever and so their bodies have become genetically able to withstand that diet.[15] (Housewife, urban Japan)

Western bodies go with Western food, but Japanese bodies do not. The implication is not that Western food is inherently bad. Rather, the Western diet is perceived as *particularly* bad for Japanese. It is, as one successful businessman put it, "ill-suited" for the Japanese body (*karada ni awanai*) and so the natural result of a westernizing diet is illness—in this case, rising rates of diabetes.

This is a logical extension of the idea that Japanese food culture and Japanese bodies co-evolved and is demonstrated in several previous quotes. When interview respondents suggested that Japanese were evolutionarily adapted to a Japanese diet, they frequently offered Western bodies and the Western diet that goes with them as another example of the same phenomenon. Junichi, the successful businessman quoted at the beginning of the chapter, followed up his claim that the Japanese body evolved to eat a meat- and fat-free diet by asking rhetorically, "In the West, people have inherited the constitution of their ancestors who ate meat from long, long ago, right?"

This question contained two interesting assumptions. The first is explicit — that early in human evolution, "at a time when people were close to monkeys," the people from whom Westerners have descended were eating meat rather than the proverbial nuts and berries of the primeval Japanese diet. The second assumption is less explicit, but perhaps even more interesting: *that Westerners do not get sick from Western diets.* Indeed, many respondents were surprised to hear that rates of diabetes were higher in the United States than in Japan. They were aware that Americans were fattened by their diet but not that they were sickened by it.

I have argued so far that lay narratives about diabetes in Japan are distinguished by several characteristics. First, they reference popular notions of evolution to explain why the Japanese body and Japanese food naturally go together. Second, these narratives generally deem Western food unhealthy for Japanese bodies, while taking for granted the actual nutritional content of everyday Japanese food. Finally, they distinguish Western bodies from Japanese bodies, positing that the Western diet is suitable for Western bodies but not for Japanese bodies.

Together, the three elements of this narrative set up a correspondence between Japanese food culture and the Japanese body on the one hand, and foreign food cultures and their corresponding bodies on the other. They suggest that it is natural for Japanese food culture and Japanese bodies to line up; when they do, diabetes is not a threat to the population. But when they do not, as in contemporary Japan, Japanese put themselves at risk. The primary model that most lay respondents rely on to make sense of the diabetes epidemic thus symbolically aligns Japanese bodies with Japanese food culture and suggests that when the two are thrown out of alignment the result is illness. The answer to the question of how to prevent or reduce the diabetes epidemic, then, is to *be more Japanese.*

Biomedical Professional Narratives

Japanese physicians and co-medicals are not insulated from this model by way of their professional training or commitment to science, just as American physicians and co-medicals are not insulated from the most common discourses surrounding diabetes in North America. In interviews, during examinations, at diabetes education seminars, and in informal conversation, Japanese physicians and co-medicals offered their own narratives of Japan's diabetes epidemic, which mirror and reify the same symbolic alignment of Japanese food culture and Japanese physiology present in lay explanations.

Professional narratives about the origins and causes of diabetes are more complex than lay narratives in large part because respondents with biomedical backgrounds have much more detailed knowledge of the disease and its biomedical etiology. But professional narratives also differ because the same individual may strategically employ several different approaches to explaining the disease to different patients, and these approaches may differ from the ways in which he or she thinks about the disease personally. The physicians and other medical professionals who graciously allowed me into their lives are by and large health *care* professionals, not researchers or professors. The majority of their work consists of real patient contact—internists in both the suburban and urban outpatient clinics saw as many as thirty patients in a single morning. Most of these doctors, nurses, and nutritionists took a pragmatic approach to presenting diabetes to their patients, switching between approaches according to what they believed would work with each patient.

These pragmatic professional narratives are the narratives I examine here. I do not attempt to discern the interior or "real" belief of the medical professionals who agreed to participate in this study if and when they offer multiple explanations of the disease. The fact that medical professionals switch between multiple narrative approaches is evidence of professional fluency, not an attempt to conceal "real" feelings. In this chapter, I analyze the narratives they present to patients and to me as explanations that are at least as professional and strategic as they are personal.

Provider narratives about type 2 diabetes contain many of the same elements as lay narratives. First, they reference a shared primordial past *specific to Japanese* in order to explain Japanese susceptibility to the disease, mixing broad evolutionary explanations with explanations of individual genetic risk. Second, while they problematize the notion that all Japanese food is good for Japanese bodies to a greater degree than lay narratives, they share a preoccupation with the importance of returning to traditional Japanese food culture. This element leads to a key difference in food recommendations for Japanese patients: white rice, anathema to diabetes patients in the United States, is a daily part of the recommended diet for Japan's type 2 diabetes patients. Finally, biomedical narratives about the origins of the diabetes epidemic contrast the lifestyle of contemporary Japan with that of the traditional *furusato*, or hometown village.

Referencing the Primordial Past, Mixing Genetics and Evolution

Health care providers, like laypeople, referenced a primordial past, in which Japanese bodies and Japanese food co-evolved, in order to explain the risk for diabetes to patients. In interviews and explanations to patients in exam rooms and diabetes classrooms, they connected individual genetic predisposition to a simplified account of human evolution in which Japanese bodies came to be distinct from others. Health care professionals tell their patients that Japanese, having evolved in a particular environmental context associated with a particular diet, are genetically predisposed to type 2 diabetes. While this narrative is more nuanced than that offered by lay respondents, it mirrors the symbolic alignment of Japanese bodies and Japanese food culture common to lay narratives and couches a cultural origin story in technoscientific language through reference to the Japanese genome.

First, providers closely connected genetic predisposition, the evolution of the Japanese people, and Japanese food. Dr. Naka, a bilingual endocrinologist at a large urban hospital, explained in a hodgepodge of Japanese and English:

> [Japanese] are prone to diabetes. Long ago, Japanese people didn't eat sweets and meat, so insulin wasn't so necessary. For more than thousands [of years] Japanese people took rice, and so insulin secretion wasn't necessary. Then after World War II, we began to eat meat and sweets. Now they need more insulin, but they don't secrete insulin to meet that [need]. Compared to Americans and Europeans, Japanese get diabetes much more easily.[16] (Endocrinologist, urban welfare hospital)

Dr. Naka says he presents this accessible explanation to patients several times a week. He suggests that, until the postwar period, the Japanese body was adapted to the Japanese diet. As new foods requiring more insulin secretion entered the Japanese diet, however, bodies no longer matched the foods they were consuming. The insulin secretion required for rice, which has a glycemic index close to that of pure honey, is left out of the story entirely.

Other health professionals' descriptions of rising diabetes rates focus on Japanese as a distinct genetic community, not on global change leading to a global rise in diabetes rates as the American narratives suggest. The explanation of risk that these health professionals offer their patients is particularistic; the idea that Japanese are physiologically unique and adapted to Japanese food is reified rather than challenged. Physicians and nutritionists saw this narrative as a way of releasing their patients from the sense that the disease is their own fault.

INTERNIST, SUBURBAN PRIVATE HOSPITAL: [High risk for diabetes] is because of the thrifty genotype. We are from our origins an island nation, and so we have a thrifty genotype that allows us to withstand not eating. I have it too. People who could withstand not eating survived.

INTERVIEWER: Do you explain the genetic component to your patients?

INTERNIST: Yes. And I explain it even for gout and hyperuricemia. For hyperlipidemia, too. There are a lot of different types of patients, but the patient who thinks, "I am just bad," is pretty common. But it's not that the patient is bad. There is a genetic component too.[17]

Explaining genetically patterned risk for diabetes and connecting it to the shared evolutionary history of the Japanese nation becomes a way to comfort patients who experience their illness as a personal failure. Referencing Japanese origins (*motomoto*) and nationality discursively moves the patient's illness from the realm of the individual to that of the community. Physicians, nurses, and nutritionists working with type 2 diabetes patients use this strategy to encourage self-deprecating patients and shift emphasis away from alienating narratives of personal responsibility.

The Preoccupation with Japanese Food Culture

Health care providers typically associated the recent upsurge in type 2 diabetes with the popularity of non-Japanese food, rather than changing ways of consuming Japanese food. Many medical professionals single out Western food in particular. Japanese food, on the other hand, was described as basically healthy. Even with the contemporary tendency to overeat, participants suggested, Japanese food could not be unhealthy and thus not the source of the diabetes epidemic:

INTERVIEWER: Why do you think rates of diabetes have been rising in Japan recently?

HEAD NURSE, SUBURBAN PRIVATE HOSPITAL: I think there is a relationship between that and dietary habits (*shokushukan*). Um, it must be dietary habits. It's fairly, well . . . obesity. Eating too much. Yes, it's because people eat an incredible amount. And Japanese food—if you eat Japanese food it's fine. Japan's food is good, but things from foreign countries like hamburgers . . . well . . . [18]

While the head nurse acknowledges that contemporary Japanese eating habits are characterized by overeating, she does not see Japanese-style food as the real source of the problem. Rather, it is the overconsumption of foreign foods that precipitates disease.

Beyond suggesting that Japanese food is less dangerous than foreign foods, even in large quantities, the providers evidenced a preoccupation with traditional foods. Health professionals qualified their endorsement of Japanese food more carefully than lay respondents, but still emphasized that the best way to prevent diabetes was to return to traditionally Japanese food. While Western food was only described as safe in small portions, Japanese food was identified as generally good.

It's good if you can have a balance like Japanese food, but no matter how hard [my clients] try, they use oil to cook.[19] (Nutritionist, urban hospital)

Japanese food is contrasted to non-Japanese food, which is frequently described as oily. Like in the lay sample, physicians and co-medicals mixed references to Japanese diet in with discussions of healthy diet. In the process, Japanese food is marked as healthy and foreign food is dubbed unhealthy, sometimes with little regard to actual nutritional content. Japanese food, unlike foreign food, is imagined to be prepared with little cooking oil and low in sugar.

The sense that Japanese bodies evolved alongside Japanese food, and that the traditional Japanese diet is well suited to Japanese bodies, contributes to a dietary recommendation that is strikingly different from those found in the United States: Japanese physicians, co-medicals, and diabetes literature aimed at patients regularly recommend white rice as part of a balanced diabetes diet. In the United States, white rice is ruled out of most recommended diets for diabetes patients due to its high glycemic index and status as a refined carbohydrate. A Harvard public health study seems to support this practice (or prejudice, depending on one's perspective), finding that individuals consuming 150 grams of rice five or more times per week were at an elevated risk for type 2 diabetes (Sun et al. 2010). The same year, a prospective cohort study in Japan confirmed the association between rice consumption and risk for diabetes, at least for women (Nanri et al. 2010).

In Japan, however, white rice is part of a balanced diet for diabetes patients and the Japan Diabetes Society recommends that patients get 50 to 60 percent of their calories from carbohydrates (JDS 2016). Diabetes education materials providing pictures of balanced meals frequently include bowls of rice, and physicians and nutritionists include it in their dietary recommendations. One diabetes specialist interviewed at a prestigious national medical center said that he recommends his type 2 diabetes patients eat 150 grams of rice per day. When I hesitated, he laughed. "You're surprised, aren't you?"

he asked. For type 1 diabetes patients, he said, he encourages "carb counting." But for type 2 patients, he says he has never recommended rice restrictions and never will. It is all a question of balance, he explained, and "rice is the backbone" (*chushin*) of the balanced Japanese diet. He went on to say of Japanese food:

> I think rice and fish are fundamental and good. And of course I think it's good to reduce oil.[20] (Diabetologist, urban national medical center)

Because rice is fundamental to the Japanese diet, it cannot be bad. Rather, the rise of a diabetes epidemic in Japan is more easily blamed on the proliferation of oil—a hallmark of westernization.

Carbohydrate intake in Japan is substantially higher than in the United States, but its content is very different. In Japan, 57 percent of energy intake comes from carbohydrates, but the most common source is rice (Sato et al. 2017a; MHLW 2014). By comparison, in the United States, 49 percent of calories come from carbohydrates, but the most common source is soft drinks (14 percent) (Sato et al. 2017a; NHANES). Only 3 percent of carbohydrate intake in America is from rice or cooked grains (Sato et al. 2017a; NHANES).

For the most part, the diabetology community in Japan has not embraced low-carbohydrate diets for reducing progression of impaired glucose tolerance and type 2 diabetes. While such diets have gained more proponents in recent years (Yamada 2017), even in early 2018 calorie-reduction diets remained the only formally recognized dietary intervention in Japan. Most providers say that while it may be useful for a small number of patients, it is not appropriate for most.

Recently, there has been more evidence of interest in carbohydrate reduction in Japan, including efforts to test and offer lower-carbohydrate diets to patients living with diabetes. A randomized controlled trial comparing a diet reducing carbohydrate consumption to 130g/day to the Japan Diabetes Society recommended calorie restriction diet found temporary improvements in glycemic control among the patients who reduced carbohydrates (Sato et al. 2017a). However, most patients randomized to the intervention arm found the 130g/day goal impossible to accomplish or sustain. Moreover, the effect disappeared within one year, perhaps because patients returned to eating 200 or more grams of carbohydrates per day almost immediately (Sato et al. 2017b). In an attempt to reconcile interest in carbohydrate reduction with the pervasiveness of rice, others have tested a "mini" diet adaptation (Kimura et al. 2018). In this adaptation, patients were asked to restrict carbohydrate consumption during just one meal per day.

Many of the health care providers were concerned about the growing use of oil in restaurants, processed foods, and home cooking. One of the particular dangers of oil (and other non-Japanese food elements) is that its strong tastes can permanently warp the Japanese palate. A well-traveled neurosurgeon worried about changes to the Japanese diet he observed to take place during his lifetime said:

> I think it's very important to get [used] to stimulating food when [children] are young . . . If they give many greasy, oily, or salty things to their children, I think the brain will memorize those, [then] they can't satisfy them with subtle tastes. In Japan we used to have subtle-taste food . . . very subtle taste. Soup is very subtle taste. Miso soup is a bit salty, but we have many things in subtle taste—less oil, less salt . . . (Neurosurgeon, urban welfare hospital and university medical center)

A supervising ward nurse had similar concerns about the changing palate of the next generation of Japanese:

> Lately here, we have come to say that Japanese food is good, of course, but . . . there has been a shift from Japanese food culture to Western food culture. Western food culture is already becoming more common than Japanese. The younger generation, in particular, prefer Western foods to Japanese side dishes. If we're talking about children, it's hamburgers and fried shrimp and things like that. That's what they like. They like it and so that's what the parents make. Those kids get big and then the nice things about Japanese food . . . how to put it? If they just eat whatever they like without learning the charms of Japanese food, I worry that eventually they will become like that [sick with diabetes]. Japanese are a fish-eating race. But young children . . . nowadays, Japanese children like meat more than fish.[21] (Supervising ward nurse, suburban private hospital)

Changes to the Japanese diet not only cause health problems but also threaten to permanently change the way that Japanese eat. Once the next generation becomes used to "unsubtle" food, its ability to enjoy the food tradition of their parents and grandparents is endangered. Thus the neurosurgeon and nurse see cultural as well as physiological danger for Japanese in the popularization of Western food styles.

Nostalgia

Professional narratives about the origins of diabetes are not restricted to the emphasis on the loss of Japanese food culture. Providers also conjure up nostalgic images of a past Japanese lifestyle thought to have been lost to urbanization, modernization, and westernization. In diabetes education classes at both hospitals offering a diabetes curriculum, traditional *furusato* (hometown/village) culture was repeatedly contrasted to contemporary Japan in order to partially explain the rising risk of diabetes for contemporary Japanese. *Furusato* culture is depicted as simple, hard-working, and rooted in traditional Japanese values. People ate Japanese food, walked from place to place, and experienced little stress. Contemporary Japan, on the other hand, is characterized by stress, irregular eating, and dependence on cars, bicycles, and public transportation.

Even the language of these explanations invokes nostalgia; descriptions of risk factors for type 2 diabetes frequently began with the words "long, long ago" (*mukashi mukashi*), the same phrase that typically precedes folk tales. Long, long, ago Japanese were not at risk for diabetes because they enjoyed a lifestyle lost to contemporary Japan. Contemporary residents of Japan no longer eat home-style Japanese food, exercise in the course of their daily work, or enjoy low-stress lifestyles. Diabetes education materials from the suburban private hospital even include graphic representations of the contrast between the traditional Japanese lifestyle of the imagined past and contemporary lifestyle. The contemporary Japanese man at risk for diabetes is portrayed eating fried food late at night, has disordered eating patterns, faces stress from his relationship with his boss, and drives his car or rides a bicycle instead of going places on foot.

Biomedical professionals engaging in diabetes education efforts draw on this contrast to convey proper preventative behavior to patients. One endocrinologist, for example, explained the need for regular exercise by telling her class, "In old times Japanese exerted themselves (*hataraku*) a lot, but recently many people have cars and other convenient devices." Like many statements about diabetes, this one refers explicitly to Japanese. Similar to the "in old times Japanese ate such-and-such" lay narrative, the endocrinologist does not refer to modern man or citizens of wealthy nations—she narrows her statement to Japanese. But she also contrasts the current environment that causes sickness (in this case, too much convenient transportation) with an imagined traditional past to which the Japanese body is more suited—though in this case the past to which she refers is much more proximate.

By harkening back to an imagined *furusato* culture, the disruption of which is imagined to have precipitated disease and dysfunction, Japanese health professionals emphasize Japan's imagined homogeneity through shared cultural and physiological heritage. By conjuring up contrasting images of the village versus the city, foot travel versus motorized transportation, and *washoku* versus Western food, they erase the emerging class differences that may contribute to different risk profiles for different parts of the population. Instead, the emphasis is on the shared trial of (mal)adjustment to a cultural milieu that is perceived to be increasingly westernized.

One (biomedical) physician referred to traditional Chinese medicine to explain the relationship between contemporary life and diabetes:

> It's the westernization of our food lifestyle, insufficient exercise, and probably stress. Chinese medicine (*kampo*) and acupuncture say . . . when you tire easily, experience exhaustion, you have insufficient spirit (*qi/ki*). In short, your energy is insufficient. If you think of it as a battery, it's like the electrical current from the battery has been stopped. There are a lot of people who feel like this. They're tired. And, well, they get irritated, they get stressed. That's because the *qi* can't move through the whole body. The number of people for whom the *qi* is not flowing is greatly increasing. When that is the case, it's easy to get diabetes. So there are lots of people getting diabetes. They're tired. I have the impression that there are lots of people stressed and irritated, and diabetes is spreading.[22] (Internist, suburban private hospital)

Like American interviewees, medical professionals in Japan see something wrong with the contemporary society in which they practice, as evidenced by increasing numbers of people who seem to be maladapted and sick with stress—or, for that matter, at risk of being maladapted and sick. But American and Japanese respondents use different metaphors to understand the ways this illness manifests itself, different explanatory models to explain it, and are nostalgic for different sources of health and well-being. Japanese respondents—particularly medical professionals—express nostalgia for a lifestyle imagined to be more purely Japanese.

Conclusions

By considering the ways in which domestic discourses on "Japanese-ness" shape seemingly unrelated medical practices and ideas, we can observe the ways in which cultural construction and mass production of Japanese uniqueness mythology shape the lived experience of ordinary people through both the experience of illness and the imperative to maintain health. Many of these discourses on health and illness mirrored *nihonjinron* themes such as the purported uniqueness of the Japanese body, the natural pairing of Japanese bodies and Japanese food culture, and nostalgia for a lost Japanese village culture.

Locating Japanese identity politics in biomedicalized explanations of Japan's diabetes epidemic tells us something important about biomedicalization. *Nihonjinron*-inflected ideas about the Japanese body are part of respondents' cultural tool kits, drawn out when they are useful for making sense of the problem at hand, not self-conscious or closely held ideologies. Yet these cultural tools of convenience have consequences for the course of biomedicalization because they influence the social values and assumptions that biomedicalization inscribes into social practice.

Despite the ubiquity of references to evolution and adaptation (or maladaptation) in narratives about the origins of diabetes in both the United States and Japan, their symbolic uses in these narratives differ considerably. Japanese narratives of the rise of the diabetes epidemic posited a specifically Japanese body adapted to the context of a specifically Japanese culture. When the symbolic alignment between the specifically Japanese body and Japanese culture is disrupted, and the body is subjected to foods and practices to which it is not adapted, the result is illness.

Both lay respondents and medical professionals used the concept of evolution to connect modern day diabetes risk to a distant past they described as uniquely Japanese. The evolutionary explanatory mechanism they used to explain diabetes risk is not applicable to all humans adjusting to industrialized realities. Rather, the concept of evolution was used to suggest that Japanese are physiologically unique from the rest of the world. Respondents explained risk using a concept that seems to be universal — evolution — but wielded it in the service of much more local ways of understanding the world. The seemingly universal, globalized language of science and medicine is thus used to express profoundly local concerns with Japanese identity and the perils of globalization.

This analysis also supports and presses Clarke's (2010: 104) assertion that "things medical" are at least partly co-constitutive with the iconography of popular culture. Clarke writes, "'[T]hings medical' . . . are not only accompanied by and reflected in popular cultural iconography — multiple media — but also were and continue to be generated and produced by and through them" (32). The present chapter deals not with literal iconography but with the conventional symbolism of the Japanese body in contemporary Japan. But the conclusion is similar: "things medical" are not only the source material for popular depictions of Japanese identity—popular depictions of Japanese identity shape and even create "things medical" in the Japanese context.

BIOMEDICALIZATION THEORY EMPHASIZES transformations and movement. Looking to Japan reminds us that it is also not a framework that over-determines: transformations of biomedical knowledge, practice, co-optation, and challenge do not follow a set path in every context. Rather, the very dynamism of biomedicalization interacts with its contexts to create myriad possibilities and probabilities. If we look away from the familiar U.S. context, we see biomedicalization reinscribing different assumptions into social practice.

One consequence of this difference is that the implied moral imperative to manage risk is also constructed differently—shaping how patients with diabetes are assessed by their health care providers. The next two chapters explore related differences in the assessment of diabetes patients by physicians in the United States and Japan, and how these different assessments lead to differences in the care offered to such patients.

CHAPTER FOUR

Your Diabetes

U.S. Health Care Providers' Orientations toward Patients

> I don't manage your diabetes. You manage your diabetes.
> —Registered nurse, certified diabetes educator

I met Rachel Frassen, an endocrinology fellow at a prestigious medical center, for coffee in a hospital food court on a sunny winter afternoon. Dr. Frassen radiated energy and purpose as she described her packed schedule of research and practice across three local medical centers and a free clinic. Like her fellow younger physicians and nurse practitioners, she emphasized her commitment to less paternalistic, "patient-centered" medicine, especially for managing chronic conditions like diabetes. But as she shifted from her belief in the merits of patient-centered care to the realities of her practice, she caught herself.

"Things need to be individualized and people need to make their own decisions and doctors aren't allowed to be paternalistic," Dr. Frassen rattled off mechanically, with a note of irony. "And people here do not respond well to paternalistic," she continued before pausing suddenly. "No, I take that back. Some people respond well to paternalistic doctoring, and other people do not, and I think it's something that—not having a ton of experience I am already starting to sort of get the hang of who needs to be told, and the vets at the VA need to be told."

It comes as no surprise that different providers have different bedside manners. What may be a surprise to some, though, is that the same providers have different bedside manners with different patients. Physicians' and nurse practitioners' interaction styles may say more about how they assess the needs of the patient than about their own philosophy of patient care. An older veteran, providers say, might prefer to be given clear instructions, while a younger lawyer might prefer a more participatory role in managing his diabetes. Providers, in effect, find themselves trying to manage their patients into managing the disease.

Though the patient management strategies they end up embracing differ, both American and Japanese providers report socially assessing their type 2 diabetes patients and tailoring their own practice to those assessments.

Learning to manage interactions with patients is a critical part of medical professionalization in almost any context. Hearing what patients are trying to say, anticipating what they want from their provider, managing their expectations, and motivating them to initiate or maintain health maintenance regimens are all necessary exam room skills for providers working with chronic disease patients. Research has shown that these are not easy skills to teach (Clark & Gong 2000). Instead, the strategies providers employ to evaluate and respond to their patients largely rest on tacit knowledge: implicit understandings of "what works" that emerge within particular organizational and social settings. The highly local nature of tacit knowledge accounts, at least in part, for the significant cross-national differences I describe in providers' patient management strategies.

Provider assessments of patients, strategies, and the orientations that underlie them can profoundly shape patient experiences of chronic disease, but they have been little explored. Further, the strategies that health care providers use to elicit cooperation and "compliance" are necessarily inflected by culture and context. But to what degree to they vary cross-nationally? How do providers frame diabetes to their patients in the United States and Japan? Do differing strategies affect their patients' orientation toward their illness? Might these strategies have public health implications?

This chapter examines U.S. health care providers' orientations toward their type 2 diabetes patients through their interactions with patients, strategies for patient motivation and management, and attitudes toward type 2 diabetes itself. In this chapter and the next, I argue that both American and Japanese medical professionals switch between different models of the provider-patient relationship as they see fit given the patient and situation at hand. This is an essentially pragmatic approach to negotiating with patients in an effort to elicit cooperation and participation in their own self-management. Practitioners in both contexts also share a belief in the power of medicalizing lifestyle recommendations to reduce stigma and improve adherence, consciously relying on medical authority to "sell" behavioral changes to some patients.

But there is one cross-national difference in orientation and strategy with potentially important consequences: the management of expectations. In sharp contrast to the Japanese providers in the next chapter, the American health care providers in this chapter described consciously monitoring and depressing their own expectations of patients. This reflects underlying differences in the way that health care providers think and talk about diabetes, and has implications for the character of diabetes care in each country.

This chapter presents and discusses three patterns in the American practitioners' conversations about treating type 2 diabetes. First, practitioners describe their efforts to take a patient-centered, rather than paternalistic, approach to treating their patients, reflecting trends in research on diabetes treatment and better patient-provider interactions. This is hardly surprising and will come as good news to many, but the interview data suggest that the reality of patient-centered approaches is more troubling than it first seems. In the name of participatory medicine, more and more moral responsibility for health is shifted to the individual patient. Second, providers approach their own medical authority as one tool among many, play-acting at old-fashioned paternalistic practice when they believe it will be therapeutically effective for a particular patient but playing it down when they believe it may be an impediment for changing patient behavior.

Finally, and critically, the U.S. health care providers voice remarkably low expectations of their patients' ability to manage their condition, continually returning to the idea that successful long-term diabetes management is a serious challenge even under the best of circumstances. As providers point out again and again, their diabetes patients are typically not living in circumstances likely to support sustained lifestyle change. In contrast to the Japanese providers in the next chapter, American providers are deeply pessimistic about the course of type 2 diabetes and the chances of good outcomes for type 2 diabetes patients.

Paternalism and Patientism

In interviews, the U.S.-based health professionals ritualistically referred to a past in which American medical practice was paternalistic and organized around doctors rather than patients. Providers said paternalistic medicine was built on a hierarchical authority structure that is no longer sound. In this supposedly outdated style of medical practice, the doctor (or other medical professional) ordered and the patient followed. By and large, respondents felt that this style of practice no longer characterized the majority of American medical practice, though its last, stubborn vestiges were frequently cited as sources of frustration. While none of the health care providers interviewed described their own practice style as paternalistic, the majority described witnessing paternalistic practices among other providers, usually physicians.

Providers universally described the shift away from paternalism, and the punitive approach associated with it, as a good thing. The hierarchical, one-way relationship that paternal practice demanded of patients left them cold. While interviewees acknowledged that this style of practice remains prevalent especially among a "certain generation" of physicians, not a single respondent identified their own personal styles with paternalism. This is perhaps partly because 65 percent of respondents were nurse practitioners trained in a tradition that has historically emphasized a patient-centered approach, rather than the medical education tradition. Even as the nursing profession becomes more specialized (and many nurse practitioners can cite as many years of education as their physician counterparts), it remains rooted in a patient-centered philosophy of care (Judd et al. 2009). Nurse practitioners and physicians alike told stories of colleagues who engaged in paternalistic practices, but without exception the subjects of these anecdotes were medical doctors.

More than simply not being interested in treating patients that way themselves, respondents argued, paternalist approaches just would not work with most of their patients. Anecdotes about paternalistic colleagues almost always had the same moral:

> [At grand rounds] the subject got onto obesity or weight management or whatever, and one of these older docs came in saying, "Well, if they would just do what I told them to do . . ." There are some older people that have a very paternalistic view of the provider-patient relationship and that they're supposed to just, you know, do everything that you tell them to do. *And if you look at the psychology behind that, that's not how it works when you're working with adults.* (Nurse practitioner [emphasis mine])

The American providers argued that treating patients like children did not yield results. Every respondent from a nursing tradition and most of those from medical traditions saw demands as simply ineffective—the primary criticism of the old-fashioned provider-patient relationship was that it does not motivate most patients to make the changes required to manage their condition. Younger health care providers' opposition to paternalistic medicine was not so much philosophical or ethical, then, as pragmatic.

Worse, when the patient is uncooperative or "noncompliant," paternalistic practice can turn punitive and rely on scare tactics. Respondents identified older physicians practicing paternalistic medicine as the main source of negative feedback and scare tactics among type 2 diabetes patients. One nurse practitioner said that in the beginning of her career treating diabetes, she worked closely with a cardiac surgeon. The surgeon would enter the room, announce to the patient that if he did not lose 100 pounds he would die, and then leave the nurse practitioner to deal with the aftermath. A second nurse practitioner described the problems that arise when paternalistic practitioners try to treat type 2 diabetes patients:

> NURSE PRACTITIONER: Instead of saying "What can we do so that you can do this?" or "What can we do that's realistic?" or "How can I make—get you to get all of your insulin today?" they just go "Well, if you don't do it, you're going to have a heart attack. You're going to end up on dialysis. You're going to be blind. You'll lose your toes," that kind of thing. So I just think that's part of it.
>
> INTERVIEWER: And patients don't respond to that by—
>
> NURSE PRACTITIONER: Well, they *cry*.

Inevitably, paternalistic practitioners were frustrated by their patients' seeming inability or unwillingness to follow orders. Frustration leads to threats, and threats are seen to further undermine the patient's ability to play an active role in their own recovery or disease management. They cry, but they don't get better.

The providers unanimously agreed that threats, "negative language," and scare tactics did not lead to successful outcomes for patients with type 2 diabetes, mirroring the dominant narrative in empirical health literature. As with paternalism more generally, criticism of scare tactics focused on their inefficacy rather than on ethical concerns. "Scaring people to death is not going to get them," explained a certified diabetes educator and nurse. "All it's going to get them to do is cover their ears or pretend it doesn't exist." In addition to being nasty, providers argued, yelling at patients is simply counterproductive

Because their dislike for paternalism did not stem from ethical concerns, even practitioners who described distaste for paternal style medical practice reported using it as a strategy when they *do* think it will be effective. The young endocrinology fellow mentioned at the beginning of this chapter, for example, felt that while using negative language is never effective, embracing her authority as a medical professional and giving orders is an effective strategy with certain patients. Thus, while she accepts in theory that American doctors are no longer supposed to encourage paternalistic relationships with patients, her actual practice is ecumenical. This reliance on multiple strategies rather than strict adherence to patient-centered medicine is discussed in detail the next section.

Still, the vast majority of interviewees described using a patient-centered approach in their interactions with patients. Patient-centered, participatory approaches are their default interaction style with patients. In particular, ideas about lifestyle changes must come from the patient:

> [The patient] will go say, "I guess my children are all overweight. Maybe I should do something about that." I say—my favorite line is "I think you're on to something. I think you're on to something." Almost no matter what they say, I think they're on to something. (Nurse practitioner)

By allowing ideas about necessary lifestyle changes to originate from the patient first, health providers reasoned, the resulting advice would be more applicable to patients' particular needs, improving its likelihood of success. Encouraging patients to brainstorm involved them in their treatment and improved the chances that they would cooperate with whatever plan was settled upon. Further, it prevents provider assumptions or missteps that could endanger the patient-provider relationship.

The shift from physician-centered to patient-centered treatment profoundly changes not only the tone of the exam room encounter, but the entire approach to managing chronic disease. In this model, type 2 diabetes patients must be given the tools to self-manage their own disease, and then coaxed, coached, and wheedled along by their unrelentingly positive provider. Rather than telling the patient what to do, the provider must educate the patient about the disease and then elicit ideas from which to design treatment strategies. This approach dramatically recasts the health professional as support staff, placing the patient at the center of his or her own disease management.

> It's better, but I think we have a ways to go because the old—well, when I was in nursing school the doctor model, the medical model, was the doctors told you what to do, and the patient just did it. You know what I'm saying? So I think now this whole team model is in vogue and empowering people to take responsibility. I think we had to. I don't think that there is any other way to do it with chronic disease. If you want outcomes, if you want people to do better, they do have to take some responsibility. A medical team by itself cannot do it. The patient has a responsibility and a role, and it's our job to support them. (Registered nurse, certified diabetes educator)

This new model of the provider-patient relationship rests on two moral assumptions. First, the patient—not the health care provider—has the right to direct his care. *But also, the patient — not the health care provider — bears ultimate moral responsibility for managing his own health.*

In this model, the provider cheers from the sidelines. Health providers working with type 2 diabetes patients frequently made an analogy to "coaching" to describe this sort of relationship with patients. They give advice and provide the occasional motivational speech, but in the end it is up to the patient to self-motivate and self-manage. According to the nurse and diabetes educator quoted above, in practical terms this means,

> We're just very positive. We're very upbeat. We just say, "I don't manage your diabetes. You manage your diabetes. I see you for small windows of time, a couple of times a year, and the same for your provider. And we don't live your life twenty-four hours a day, so our job is to make sure that you have the most current up-to-date information and understand why we make the recommendations and decisions that we do about your treatment because the hard choices are going to come, well, it's always after 5:00 on a Friday night and your doctor is not on call, or they're out of town. So we want you to be the best informed consumer about you." (Registered nurse, certified diabetes educator)

The medical team can't accompany the patient twenty-four hours a day. In the American health care system, they can't even see most patients more than twice a year. Empowering patients to take an active role in managing type 2 diabetes is imperative when they have relatively little contact with health practitioners.

Giving patients a sense of control may be particularly important for managing type 2 diabetes. Women and men with chronic illness confront depression at a higher rate than the general population (Ford 2008), and many others experience depressive symptoms that do not meet the criteria for major depressive disorder (Gonzalez et al. 2011), or a generalized sense of defeat or failure (Charmaz 1991). People with type 2 diabetes have a particularly high rate of depression: more than 50 percent of patients present with comorbid major depression (American Diabetes Association 2007), so many that some providers that participated in this study report prescribing antidepressants to patients immediately upon their initial diabetes diagnosis. At least one major meta-analysis suggests that the presence of depression may be a risk factor for developing type 2 diabetes, rather than the other way around (Mezuk et al. 2008). Many patients suffer from depression before they are diagnosed with type 2 diabetes, and their diagnosis may exacerbate their depression (Mezuk et al. 2008). In addition to managing a chronic disease that may require changes to every part of their lifestyle, type 2 diabetes patients may be blamed for their disease by strangers, friends, family, and even some of their own health care providers. The barrage of negative assessments can eat away at patients' sense of self worth and further impair their ability to make positive lifestyle changes or even function in daily life.

For people labeled as having "my-fault diabetes," facing stigma and depression, patient empowerment approaches promise to be transformative. In theory, the patient-centered "empowerment" approach involves patients in their own care, cultivates independence, and gives them the opportunity to develop confidence and control over some aspect of their lives. When patients are empowered, the theory goes, they can feel that they are making decisions for themselves and see that the changes they make result in a better quality of life. Providers argued that this can start a cycle of positive feedback that leads to lasting change and improved diabetes management.

But the embrace of patient empowerment also shifts responsibility for managing the disease even further to the individual patient. The old paternalistic model of medicine may have restricted patient autonomy and created a power dynamic that makes contemporary patients and practitioners uncomfortable, but it also clearly defined the responsibilities of all involved. Patients were charged with following orders, but physicians were charged with managing the well-being of their patients. In contrast, contemporary health care providers operating with a patient-centered model of care remind themselves to define their own responsibilities more carefully:

> I think you get frustrated with the patients, but you also get frustrated seeing how their health deteriorates as a result of the disease and of the choices that they make. I think also people take on some kind of a sense of responsibility with them, and I think that you have to realize that in the end your responsibility is to educate them and to offer them the right therapies and to provide them with good medicine, to practice safe, good medicine with them and to help them make the right choices. But it's their choice. You can't save the world. (Nurse practitioner)

While interview respondents were deeply committed to their patients, they also constantly distanced themselves from bearing too much responsibility for patient well-being. They emphasized that successful disease management depends on the *patient*, not the health care provider. Patient well-being is recast as the result of patient choices, not the quality of their health care or their health care provider.

In some cases the rhetoric of patient empowerment seems more focused on emphasizing that the responsibility for the disease and its management rests with the patient than on the responsibility of the practitioner to involve the patient in his or her own care. An experienced nurse practitioner described the difference between a patient who was easy to treat and a patient who was difficult to treat in terms of their willingness to be empowered:

> Well, the ones that are easier for me to work with are willing to get control of their diabetes, and they're not defeated. The other ones are very . . . they're not really motivated, and the world is horrible, and their life is horrible, and they just can't get on top of it even though I again offered to be accessible. And then once you empower them, they *still* won't do it. (Nurse practitioner)

Here "empowerment" seems little different from a rhetoric of personal responsibility. Medical anthropologists have linked the emphasis on self-care in the treatment of type 2 diabetes in the United States with a neoliberal logic of personal responsibility and consequences (Ferzacca 2000). The linking of self-discipline, individual-level responsibility, and health creates a powerful value system internalized by patients as well as professional practitioners, and this logic may actually produce, rather than destabilize, hybrid and "idiosyncratic" self-care regimes that medical professionals tend to label as "noncompliant" or non-adherent (Ferzacca 2000). In the quote above, patient empowerment is cast as a patient *responsibility* rather than a right. This provider was frustrated with patients who, even after she goes to great lengths to make herself accessible and empower them, refuse take on this responsibility. The statement "Once you empower them, they still won't do it" betrays a sense that, at least in practice, patient empowerment approaches are founded on an assumption that patients are personally, morally responsible for their own illness and its eventual outcome. This emphasis on self-management and responsibility in American clinical discourse on diabetes can serve to continually reassert the individual as the only unit of analysis that matters (Ferzacca 2000; Broom & Whittaker 2004). Biomedical perspectives on diabetes in the United States thus reify the concept of individual health, at the cost of relational or social conceptualizations of health more common among laypeople (Loewe & Freeman 2000).

Multiple Strategies

When asked to speak in concrete terms and experiences, providers often explained that the same strategy that works wonders with one patient is liable to end in disaster with another. For example, while interviewees described VA patients as responsive to paternalistic orders and advice, patients of low socioeconomic status with no military background were frequently characterized as resistant to authority, even when the "orders" are clearly in their own best interest. The endocrinology fellow quoted earlier cautions:

> At our indigent care clinic on _____ Road, having authority is . . . you might as well put on a police uniform when going there. It's just like people are just not going to respond well to you. That's a lot more "What do you think you need to do? These are your choices." And if you ever say what you're leaning toward, then it's like my toddler. They're like "Oh, I want to do the other thing." (Physician, endocrinology fellow)

In the same week, then, this fellow may order one patient to reduce his soda intake and log his blood glucose more often but ask another patient what *he* wants to do to deal with his diabetes.

Successful treatment of type 2 diabetes requires patient cooperation and even enthusiasm, which are not always easy characteristics to elicit from patients facing chronic illness and multiple comorbid conditions. If paternalism does not work with low-income patients, health care providers consciously shift their language and recommendations to avoid negative encounters. If providers assume or sense that another population is responsive to being ordered around, they shift their language and recommendations again. Importantly, even providers who reported having a particular philosophy of practice also reported relying on multiple styles of practice depending on the patient in question. This is congruent with conversation analyses of patient-provider interactions and clinical decision-making exercises that find providers focus on patients' cognitive and psychosocial characteristics first (Lutfey et al. 2008).

Many diabetes patients blame themselves for their condition, just as many are blamed by those around them. The association with obesity only exacerbates the stigma of what some patients call "my-fault diabetes." Sensitive health care providers recognize that many patients, especially female patients, are embarrassed by their condition and by the recommendation to lose weight. Because providers agreed that scaring and shaming patients into lifestyle changes did not work, they were eager to show patients that they were not judging them.

> It's easy to sort of, I think, approach a weight loss discussion by offering these medical things. It takes away the stigma a little bit for people because what I'm saying is not "You look ugly" but "I think this would be good for your health." . . . I think one of the important things about obesity counseling and type 2 diabetes counseling is setting goals and writing them down and then giving people specific tasks, like I want you to—I give prescriptions for things like "I want you to eat so and so calories a day" or I write them a prescription to cut down on sodas, and sometimes I feel like again like medicalizing it a little bit to try to take the stigma away. (Endocrinologist)

This endocrinologist believed that writing lifestyle prescriptions emphasizes two points to her patients. First, her weight loss recommendations do not come from a personal evaluation of her patient; they arise from her professional training as a doctor. She said she even makes a point of telling many of her female patients that they look beautiful just how they are, but that if they want to treat their diabetes they must start a weight loss plan. Explicitly separating personal evaluations from professional evaluations, and cosmetic evaluations from medical evaluations, helps her to cut through the shame and confusion patients may experience when confronted with weight loss.

Second, writing prescriptions for lifestyle behavior lends gravity to daily behaviors that may otherwise seem unimportant to patients. Writing a prescription gives medical authority to the recommendation to cut out soda or walk to the mailbox three times per day. Without the prescription, patients are likely to believe that taking the oral medication for their type 2 diabetes is more important than walking to the mailbox. One of the ways the endocrinologist can signal to patients that diet and exercise are as important as pharmacological interventions is by writing a prescription for one just as they would the other. Just as providers sometimes play-act at giving paternalistic orders, they also work to medicalize lifestyle recommendations.

Health care providers are essentially pragmatic in the exam room; all respondents reported using a variety of strategies depending on the patient and context. They consciously perform multiple, seemingly contradictory forms of medical authority, sometimes over the course of a single encounter. This means that while most providers describe their practice as patient-centered and criticize outdated "paternalistic" approaches to the provider-patient relationship, they also use more paternalistic strategies when they think it will suit the patient.

Grim Expectations

Providers took the call to shift from compliance to adherence (Lutfey & Wishner 1999) seriously. They consistently framed adherence within the context of patient social settings and resources. Doing so added substantial complexity to their clinical decision making. Most sympathized deeply with their patients. Several described the emotional labor associated with simultaneously assessing and responding to patients and their social circumstances.

Perhaps what is most striking about American providers' discussions of diabetes in interviews, though, is their overwhelming pessimism. Even as they described patient-centered empowerment approaches to patient care, the health care providers interviewed voiced relatively low expectations of their patients. Even as they said that their approach was unrelentingly positive, in private they were often profoundly pessimistic on the topic of patient prospects. While Japanese physicians expected a high degree of self-discipline from their patients, and became concerned when they did not exhibit the hoped-for degree of discipline, American practitioners repeatedly cautioned that expectations should be low for significant subsets of their patient populations. Health providers say they remind themselves that "people who go to [the free clinic are usually] people who don't search for opportunity themselves," that "people just can't count," and that it is most productive to just "commend them on whatever they are able to do."

There is some evidence supporting this lack of confidence in patients' willingness or ability to follow medical advice. U.S.-based studies have shown that even when patients are asked to self-report on their own adherence to the simplest instructions from their providers—to take one oral medication once or twice a day—more than 15 percent say they do not consistently take their diabetes medications (Cerimagic 2004). But providers generally did not refer to these studies to justify their lack of confidence in patients' ability and subsequent low expectations.

Rather, providers connect low expectations to their sympathy with the difficulties that patients faced. A primary care physician whose practice encompassed patients from a variety of socioeconomic backgrounds described how he controlled his own expectations of his patients:

I try to remember especially for my patients who, like I said, whose social environment is a mess so any progress they would make would have to be them completely going against the grain of everything they've ever known and everything going on in their life, and so I do feel a little bit, you know, I do feel kind of sorry for those people because, like I said, those people who have very limited food options it's hard to imagine what kind of effort that would take to make that level of change. (Primary care physician)

This provider cited neither disdain nor the empirical literature, but rather his own assessment that the economic and cultural environments of his patients do not support successful diabetes management.

Clinical decision making is a complex, multidimensional process in which providers amalgamate clinical, epidemiological, and psychosocial assessments. The first and most important of these assessments may be psychosocial. Lutfey et al. (2008) found that physicians engage in complex assessment with little reference to epidemiologic profiles. In controlled, vignette-based factorial experiments, physicians in the U.S. and the U.K. first assessed the cognitive skills of the patient, then assessed social support (Lutfey et al. 2008). In "thinking out loud" to reach a diagnostic and treatment decision, physicians mentioned patients' cognitive and psychological traits more frequently than either physical symptoms or epidemiologically relevant demographic characteristics (Lutfey et al. 2008). Lutfey et al. (2008) concluded that physicians may interpret practice guidelines, including base rates, in terms of behavior rather than biology.

Some of the providers felt that low expectations were probably detrimental to successful outcomes but confessed to holding low expectations privately even while treating patients as if their expectations were high.

I always like to give them the benefit of the doubt. If they're initially diagnosed with diabetes, and they want to do no medication and do diet and exercise and lifestyle changes first, I'm okay with that, but it's hard for me to believe that they're going to control their diabetes with just lifestyle and exercise. (Nurse practitioner)

Even when providers want to believe in their patients, their body of experience makes it hard to suspend their disbelief for each new patient.

Of course, it is easier to believe that some patients will bring their blood glucose under control than others. Educated, organized, "type A" patients were routinely identified as the kind of patients who could be counted on to manage their diabetes with lifestyle interventions. Practitioners' lowest expectations were of patients with less education, those facing economic challenges, and those who present with comorbid psychiatric conditions like depression. Little was expected of "Type B," easygoing personalities who are seen as lacking a sense of urgency or discipline.

Many of the providers interviewed said they simply do not want to set expectations from which their patients may derive a further sense of failure. Sometimes they explicitly cited a low estimation of patient's cognitive ability, but providers also argued that lifestyle change is challenging—and that even if a patient successfully implements change, that may only be half the battle.

> If you can monitor your blood sugar the way your provider asks you to do it, if you can take your insulin or your oral agents the way you're supposed to, and you can eat reasonably and do what you're supposed to do and add exercise . . . But you know? Some days your blood sugars are just going to beat to their own drum, and that's because only 50 percent of diabetes are things we can really do something about. The other 50 percent are counterregulatory hormones and physiological processes, but we have no access to that hormone switch. And it would be very hard to do all the right things all the time. (Registered nurse, certified diabetes educator)

Even when patients do all the right things, the most sympathetic providers pointed out, they have limited control over their bodies' physiological processes. No matter what type 2 diabetes patients do, there will be days where their blood sugar is too high. No matter what they do, eventually the disease will progress. This sense of pessimism has been noted in the few other accounts of providers' diabetes explanatory models as well (Loewe & Freeman 2000). In the interviews considered here, providers called type 2 diabetes "very, very difficult" and even unmanageable.

The perception that diabetes is essentially outside the control of provider and patient alike has inevitable consequences in the exam room. In order to protect patients from the inevitable emotional fatigue of a chronic, progressive condition like diabetes, health care providers try to set and communicate what they consider to be "realistic" expectations to their patients. These are goals that they judge their patients capable of achieving, and from which they hope that particularly defeatist patients may derive a greater sense of self-efficacy and control. The goals that providers judge their patients capable of achieving are more often than not painfully modest: common examples included cutting down their sweet tea or soda consumption by one glass per day and walking as far as the mailbox once a day. In order to achieve patients' targets for diabetes management, the providers instead relied on pharmaceutical interventions, often combining two or more medications and orienting the patient encounter around the adjustment of these medications (see Hunt, Kreiner & Brody 2012).

The providers said they hoped to cultivate a sense of control over diabetes by setting realistic expectations and attainable goals rather than by encouraging, for example, disciplined documentation on the part of the patient. While health providers said that calorie and carbohydrate counting are "really, really helpful" for patients if they are willing to keep food diaries, most did not ask their patients to do so. Instead, providers overwhelmingly preferred simple approaches deemed more realistic because they do not require numeracy or discipline. "The best diet is whatever diet you can stick with and do," explained one doctor. "One of the reasons I like [low carbohydrate diets] is they tend to have few very simple guiding principles rather than complicated calorie or carb counting in them . . . I like diets that are a little bit simpler to talk to people about."

But these "realistic expectations" are premised on providers' surprisingly fatalistic, pessimistic orientation toward the progression of type 2 diabetes. Providers use language that suggests hopelessness when they describe type 2 diabetes. Blood sugars are liable to "beat to their own drum," it is "hard to believe" it can be controlled with lifestyle and exercise, and patients attempting lifestyle change will find it "very, very difficult." Many patients' lives are characterized as "a mess," change goes "against the grain of everything they have every known," and their Type B personalities mean they "don't search for opportunity themselves." When providers see diabetes as unmanageable and their patients as unreliable managers, they settle for low expectations.

The end result was that the goals and strategies health care providers set for their patients were on a relatively small scale. They focused on small lifestyle changes—reducing soda consumption from three or four cans a day to two cans, replacing one drink a day with a diet alternative, walking to the mailbox once a day—rather than grand ones. Reasoning that something is better than nothing, they encouraged patients to make small changes with small returns. They made simple recommendations that do not require patient numeracy, or even much in the way of cooperation from either the patient or the patient's metabolic system. Grander life changes might bring about greater returns, but they would carry with them greater risk of failure. Providers concluded that small changes and an ever-growing list of medications were more reliable than changes to lifestyle.

Conclusions

I have argued in this chapter that the U.S.-based providers working with type 2 diabetes patients embraced the ideal of patient-centered medicine when speaking in the abstract, but reported a great deal of variation in their actual practice when asked about concrete experiences and situations. Thus, while providers were without exception committed in theory to the idea of patient-centered medicine, they were usually ecumenical in practice. The same doctor may change his or her style of addressing and treating patients dramatically from patient to patient or from context to context. Similarly, physicians consciously medicalized the idea of lifestyle change when they think that lending lifestyle change the weight of their own medical authority will motivate the patient.

These U.S.-based providers also had notably low expectations of their patients, and cited sympathy for the socioeconomic and metabolic challenges faced by many type 2 diabetes patients in the United States to explain their low expectations. Providers' low expectations and pessimism contributed to a preference for small, simple lifestyle changes in combination with medication rather than bold lifestyle change. They felt more comfortable orienting medical visits around adjusting or adding medications to reach targets defined by surrogate markers like HbA1c, to which patients may not relate (Yudkin, Lipska, & Montori 2011).

While decades of health locus of control research has been conducted on patients and associated with poor health outcomes, little work has been done on the health locus of control of doctors and other health care providers. The fatalistic attitudes toward the progression of type 2 diabetes evidenced in the interviews here suggest that these providers believe the course of the disease to be primarily determined by forces outside their (and possibly their patients') control. Locus of control research has contributed much to understanding why some patients respond to health recommendations and intervention plans, while others do not. An internal locus of control is associated with a more proactive approach to health and greater compliance with health care provider recommendations, while an external locus of control is associated with a more fatalistic attitude toward health (AbuSabha & Achterberg 1997; Pearlin et al. 1981). Because external locus of control places individuals at higher risk for complications as a result of noncompliance (Bush 1988) and because it is sociologically patterned, it can contribute to socioeconomic and racial disparities in health outcomes (Pearlin et al. 1981).

But the provider interviews discussed here suggest that more research must be done on providers' health locus of control, how fatalism may shape practice, and whether or not providers are transmitting these attitudes to patients. Providers' conservative expectations may protect their patients from the perceived psychological risks associated with attempting bold lifestyle changes, but they may also risk affirming patient assumptions that real change is impossible and that their condition is not within their control.

Medical visits are "sense-making" events, in which patients and providers make meaning out of problems and choose strategies to resolve them. Patient resistance to advice they find unreasonable is not antagonism and is not necessarily counterproductive. Conversation analyses have demonstrated that patient resistance can be a form of engagement in the clinical encounter (Gill, Pomerantz, & Denvir 2010; Barton et al. 2016). Thought of this way, patient resistance can be reframed as a resource for clinical decision making and management. For example, patient resistance to lifestyle advice through reference to "candidate obstacles" provides an opportunity for providers to align their advice with patient realities (Barton et al. 2016). Resistance can be productive if it stimulates an exchange in which the provider gains patient-specific insight and thus is able to reframe advice. Hesitation to "ask too much" of patients whose life-worlds providers do not understand may reduce opportunity for this productive resistance.

CHAPTER FIVE

Our Diabetes

Diabetes in the Japanese Exam Room

It was 8:40 A.M.; Dr. Saito and Nurse Kurokawa were ahead of schedule. Outpatient hours did not begin for another twenty minutes and we had already reviewed the schedule for the day and checked the electronic medical records for the first appointment of the morning. For Dr. Saito, the petite internist in charge of the hospital's new type 2 diabetes clinic, this was a rare opportunity to relax during her workday, usually packed with morning outpatient hours, afternoon inpatient service rounds, and a new diabetes education program—not to mention the endless series of meetings that are part of the reality of Japanese clinical practice.

Dr. Saito was not interested in relaxing. She checked her watch and looked at her nurse, an experienced woman at least fifteen years her senior. "I wonder if there's time to visit the dialysis center?" she asked. She had been worried about a particular hemodialysis patient all week, ever since Nurse Kurokawa told her that she had heard from the nurses staffing the dialysis center that he had been having difficulties with "self-management" (*jiko kanri*).

The three of us left the outpatient clinic. As we walked to the elevator bank, Dr. Saito explained the situation. There was some question as to whether or not the patient, Ichiro, should be admitted as an inpatient. He was undergoing dialysis three times a week and had a home nurse every morning to help him administer insulin injections. Even with these aids, however, Ichiro was not controlling his blood sugar and was thought to be a nonadherent patient. Nurses reported that he was known to eat lunch in the hospital dining hall after each dialysis treatment, where he would fill his coffee mug three-quarters of the way with coffee, then pour in creamer and sugar to the top. Further, because he lived alone, there was no way to enlist the help of a wife or daughter to manage his eating, drinking, and insulin. The best thing, Dr. Saito explained, might be to admit him so that he could spend more time at the hospital learning how to "manage" himself.

Arriving at the dialysis center, we met Ichiro. I had expected someone old or infirm, but Ichiro was middle-aged, perfectly lucid, and did not appear physically infirm beyond the usual way that dialysis patients' bodies seem tired. The visiting nurse, dialysis center nurses, and doctors had been keeping a handwritten notebook for him in a style akin to — but separate from — inpatient charts, which a nurse brought over for Dr. Saito as she consulted with the patient. Because patients receiving dialysis in Japan are required to temporarily check in to the hospital and occupy a bed, Ichiro remained prone during the entire consultation.

Dr. Saito returned to the nurses' station after her short chat with the patient. There, one of the nurses told her that a senior male physician had informally expressed concern about Ichiro's behavior. Ichiro would wander into the same dining hall used by the medical staff in order to find creamer, so many of the staff were aware of his troubling coffee condiment consumption. This seemed to make up Dr. Saito's mind; she squared her jaw and nodded her head. Ichiro would be admitted to the hospital.

Approaching Ichiro's bed again, Dr. Saito reproached him for the repeated creamer incidents using a formal speech register. The patient laughed nervously and looked down at his hands. She frowned at him. In a moment, Dr. Saito was back to her usual, cheerful demeanor. She delivered the news. "Well, let's admit you," she said. ("*Dewa, nyuuin shimashou.*")

As we left, Dr. Saito explained that Ichiro would be admitted for the sake of controlling his blood sugar, in part through diet. He would be encouraged to attend the diabetes classroom and possibly learn to better manage his blood sugar and lifestyle. I asked if he was being admitted for bad behavior. "Yes, I suppose so," she replied. "It's best to admit him because his behavior is making him more sick."

Ichiro was admitted as an inpatient explicitly because he was judged incapable of successfully managing his disease on his own, despite being literate, articulate, not suffering from known cognitive deficit or mental disorder, and not being in acute danger. In the United States, admitting a patient primarily for the purposes of education would be not only ridiculous and infeasible but likely unethical. Ichiro's Japanese medical team reasoned differently: with type 2 diabetes and advanced renal failure, Ichiro's careless consumption of calories was dangerous. If he was drinking his coffee with cream and sugar in front of doctors, what was he doing at home? If Ichiro would not take care of himself, his medical team would have to do it themselves.

Some aspects of the creamer incident seem to illustrate a paternalistic model of the provider-patient relationship like the one that American providers so abhorred in the previous chapter. But it is not quite the paternalism of generations past that led Japanese physicians to hide terminal diagnoses from patients or speak to them in registers usually reserved for children and subordinates. Dr. Saito, after all, spoke to Ichiro politely and enlisted his cooperation in the decision by using "let's" (*shimashou*). If Ichiro had outright rejected the idea, he could have avoided being admitted. And Dr. Saito is a relatively young woman, while her patient is an older man—a reversal that upsets the usual gender pattern of traditional medical practice and authority in Japan, where until very recently nearly all internists were men.

There is another notable difference between this interaction and the patient-provider interactions described in the preceding chapter on U.S. patient-provider interactions. Dr. Saito acts on the basic belief that, although her patient is experiencing acute renal failure and demonstrates little interest in "managing" his own health, it is nonetheless possible to bring his condition under control and perhaps even train him to control it himself. Concluding that her patient is unable to bring his condition under control with self-management, she resolves to manage his condition on his behalf. Rather than concluding that she can only help those who help themselves, as the American providers concluded, Dr. Saito concluded that it is her own and the hospital's responsibility to manage his behavior in the interest of managing his condition.

LIKE THEIR AMERICAN counterparts in the previous chapter, Japanese providers take a pragmatic approach to negotiating with patients in order to elicit cooperation and participation in their own self-management. They switch between different models of the provider-patient relationship as they see fit, given the patient and situation at hand. Japanese providers also recognize the power of medicalizing lifestyle recommendations when they explain treatment options to patients, self-consciously relying on medical authority to "sell" behavioral change to some patients. But while the American health care providers in the previous chapter self-consciously monitored and depressed their expectations of patients, Japanese providers embrace expectations of their patients that seem almost unreasonably high, frequently favoring lifestyle change and careful monitoring over oral medication. This critical difference in the ways that health care providers think and talk about diabetes has implications for the character of diabetes care in each country.

Health care providers in the United States and Japan work with very different patient populations and within very different institutional realities, but providers in both countries approached their interactions with patients with an air of pragmatism. Like the American providers in the preceding chapter, Japanese providers adjusted the presentation of information about diabetes and even their own self-presentation to meet the perceived needs of individual patients. With one patient, providers might be rigid and polite, with another, relaxed and informal. One patient was issued strict orders, while another was asked what he wanted to do to improve his quality of life. Even as providers in both countries described keenly felt commitments to an idealized provider-patient relationship model that empowers patients to actively participate in their own care, these same providers enacted a variety of provider-patient relationship models in practice. The content and tone of interactions between type 2 diabetes patients and their health care providers varied dramatically across context.

Models of Authority in the Japanese Exam Room

In the next three sections, I examine the mechanics of medical authority in provider-patient interactions through exam room observations and interviews with doctors and patients. Like the American providers, Japanese providers eschew a paternalistic style of medical practice that they perceive to be outdated. Instead, they pursue a patient-centered approach that emphasizes respect and patient autonomy. Also like the American respondents, Japanese providers approach their own medical authority with a pragmatic air, relying on the high social status of biomedicine and play-acting at old-fashioned paternalistic medical practice when they believe it would be therapeutically effective for a particular patient.

In sharp contrast to the attitudes evidenced by the American providers, however, Japanese physicians and nurses described and demonstrated high expectations of their type 2 diabetes patients. They were optimistic about the course of the disease for most patients. While they acknowledged that the degree of discipline required to self-manage type 2 diabetes over the long term is extraordinarily high, they demanded that discipline from most patients as a matter of course. When patients failed to meet those expectations, the Japanese providers acted in ways that would be extraordinary—even, potentially, unethical—in American settings by disciplining patients themselves.

There are notable differences in the context in which Japanese physicians, nurses, and nutritionists work compared to their American counterparts. For one, the professional mix of health care providers treating patients with type 2 diabetes varies. In Japan, physicians treat most patients themselves. Nurses have almost no autonomy, the professional category of nurse practitioner is absent, and while there were around 12,000 certified diabetes educators in the entire country during the years of my fieldwork (Kawaguchi 2007), no one at my primary field site was certified. (There are shortages of diabetes educators in both the United States and Japan; the United States has around 30,000 diabetes educators, only around half of whom are certified.)

There are also significant differences across regions, prefectures, and hospitals within Japan. The private suburban hospital I mention in this chapter, for example, took many *saishin* patients. *Saishin* means simply "return visit," but those referred to as *saishin* patients are those with a chronic condition who visit a particular doctor on a regular schedule—once every other month, once a month, or even once a week. They typically have a standing appointment with their physician on the same day and time, and so doctor and patient become regular, predictable fixtures in one another's lives. Even if most of these appointments are cursory, five-minute interactions in which the physician merely renews a prescription and chats briefly with the patient, the visits build trust and familiarity. One physician I shadowed at the suburban hospital estimated that he saw nearly eighty *saishin* patients in an average week, at least half of his total caseload.

At the urban welfare hospital less than thirty minutes away, on the other hand, set *saishin* visits were less common and spaced further apart. Physicians in the diabetes clinic there emphasized that they were simply too busy to see patients so frequently, though they agreed that the practice of checking in for a five-minute appointment was helpful and preferable to their less frequent consultations. Instead of having a regular *saishin* appointment every month, patients scheduled their next visit anew at the end of each appointment, usually for four to eight weeks later. But even at the crowded urban welfare hospital, patients successfully managing type 2 diabetes were seen by a provider approximately once in every two months.

From Ordering to Exhorting

Japanese bioethicists have long argued that the Japanese model of medical authority is qualitatively different from the American model (Hoshino 1997). But young Japanese physicians, like their American counterparts, argue that the old medical culture has largely faded. Japanese providers described their efforts to shift away from a paternalistic style of medical practice that they perceive to be outdated, preferring a patient-centered approach that emphasizes respect and patient autonomy. Dr. Saito, the physician who admitted Ichiro, once commented between exams that the "style" of Japanese medicine was once rather authoritarian. "The style of medicine was 'Do this' (~*shi nasai*)," she said in a gruff voice, imitating the tone of an older, male doctor. Patients were to respond, "'Yes, sir' (*Sou shimasu*)," she said, her tone softening and rising as she imitated the imaginary patient of the past. Nowadays, she argued, a new generation of physicians had been able to change that culture for the most part.

Although Japanese providers described patient-centeredness as a work in progress, most DM consultations aligned with the three-function model that has influenced efforts at patient-centered care in the United States. In the classic three-function model for the medical interview (Cohen-Cole 1991), the biomedical objectives of the medical interview are situated within understanding of the patients' psychosocial context, establishment of an alliance-oriented therapeutic relationship with the patient, and broad-based patient education. In the United States, only a small proportion of visits reflect this "mutual" interaction model (Heritage & Maynard 2006; Roter et al. 1997).

The most obvious evidence for providers recentering around patients is in the language they use during interactions with patients. The new language of the exam room exhorts rather than orders. Younger physicians made suggestions to their patients with varying degrees of vigor and almost never used the ~*shi nasai* form to tell patients what to do. Dr. Saito and her colleagues frequently praised patients for making progress by losing weight or controlling their blood sugar, or simply maintaining an acceptable status quo. This aligned with the best practices accepted in the United States for coaching patients with chronic disease. While the Japanese providers offered more concrete recommendations and demanded a greater degree of discipline from their patients, they also elicited ideas from patients in order to involve them in their own treatment and tailor recommendations, just like the American providers. When a patient faltered or failed to meet the goals of a previous action plan, Dr. Saito would acknowledge the failure in concerned murmurs, then exhort the patient to help come up with a new plan: "Well, let's all think together!" (*Sa, minna de isshou ni kangaemashou.*)

At the suburban hospital, respect for the patient was paramount—and the use of appropriately respectful and friendly language was considered central to expressing this respect. All hospital employees (including this author) were issued a staff handbook covering topics ranging from patient rights and disaster level designations to acceptable lipstick shades and appropriate greetings. The handbook instructed hospital staff, including physicians, to adopt the demeanor of staff at an upscale hotel or Tokyo department store in all interactions with patients. Medicine, it reminded hospital staff, is *a service industry*. And like other service industries, hospital staff must strive to use correct, formal, and respectful language in their encounters with patients. The fifty-seven-page handbook classified the most common types of interactions, offering guidelines as to what greetings and language should be used in each context.

An entire section of the handbook was dedicated to polite interactions with visitors on elevators. Hospital staff were cautioned to hold the elevator for patients and visitors, engage in polite conversation without speaking about themselves personally,[1] announce each floor as the elevator stops, then hold the door open and offer directions to disembarking patients. When we reached our floor, we were to apologetically announce our departure: "Excuse me for leaving ahead of you." (*"Osaki ni shitsurei shimasu."*) The section on elevator etiquette may explain why most clinic staff chose to use the stairs to travel between the outpatient exam rooms and the dialysis center, despite their being five floors apart.

Hospital rules required all new staff to engage in role-plays and self-quizzes designed to ensure that they speak to patients in the same formal, respectful register used to speak to superiors or honored clients. Basic handbook rules for patient interaction included:

> When you meet [a patient], bow.[2]
> Don't neglect appropriate greetings.[3]
> Learn patients' names and faces as quickly as you can.[4]
> Use *-desu* and *-masu* grammar form when you speak.[5]
> No matter how busy you are, make an effort to be gentle and womanly.[6]
> When a patient has a complaint, first formally apologize by saying, "I'm so sorry; there is no excuse." Then respond in a concrete manner. As a general rule, never argue with a patient.[7]

More than half of the basic rules outlined in the staff handbook pertained to appropriate speech registers and verbal etiquette with patients.

Public daily behavior in and around the outpatient clinics of the hospital largely conformed to the written rules. Rules about politely greeting patients and colleagues in public areas were particularly strictly observed. Anyone who was not obviously a hospital employee was wished a good morning, afternoon, or evening. Fellow hospital staff—even strangers—unfailingly exchanged singsong set phrases thanking one another for their hard work. Hallway interactions with patients were friendly but formal. The only handbook rules obviously violated on a regular basis were those pertaining to receiving traditional thank-you gifts from patients, the acceptance of which remained common among the older generation of physicians. The majority of the rules laid out in the handbook were workplace norms enforced by habit, peer pressure, and a never-ending series of staff meetings.

These rules applied equally to the resident foreign researcher. On my first day of participant observation at the main reception desk, I turned my back on the patient counter for a moment to file something, only to be immediately reprimanded. A medical clerk modeled the proper way to file papers without ever showing my back to a patient. Gradually, I learned to keep my hips angled toward the counter that a patient might approach while turning my torso eighty degrees toward the file cabinet. At lunch, the clerks joked that the practice would eventually make their back muscles permanently uneven.

Of course, it is one thing for medical clerks and nurses to behave like service industry employees, and another for doctors, who have traditionally occupied one of the highest status professional categories in Japan (Long 1987; Jansen 2002). In the section of the handbook aimed at doctors, the importance of a service mindset was reiterated, as if to remind physicians that, unlike in previous eras, the general staff rules applied to them as well. The third article in the section on the hospital doctors' basic responsibilities read:

> We humbly ask that you avoid a hierarchical atmosphere or behaving as if you are bestowing treatment upon patients in doctor-patient relationships. Be especially careful in your attitude toward patients and in the way you speak to them. Please recognize that medicine is increasingly a service industry, and keep this in mind during examinations. Please familiarize yourself with this hospital's patient bill of rights.[8]

The handbook went on to remind the medical doctors on staff that "the relationship between medical doctors and co-medicals is also changing" and that doctors must shift their attitude toward their own practice in order to effectively practice team medicine. The doctors on staff are asked to exercise "leadership" (*riidashiipu*) as the hospital worked to shift to a team approach. At weekly all-hospital meetings and doctors' meetings, the hospital president and founder—an oncologist by training—repeatedly emphasized the basic goal of creating an atmosphere in which patients could feel comfortable and in control, and in which co-medicals could contribute their expertise and professional opinions without intimidation.

All this emphasis on respectful language and the self-conscious rejection of the old-fashioned power dynamic between patient and provider suggests continuing angst over the degree to which Japanese physicians have really been able to shift to patient-centered and team approaches. While Japanese providers were intensely critical of the organization and financial state of the U.S. health care system, they spoke admiringly of American leadership in developing patient-oriented and team-based practice models. In contrast, they portrayed Japan as working hard to adopt these approaches rather than fostering them independent of the American model.

Informally, though, Japanese providers pointed out that many patients did not *want* a "patient-centered" exam room experience. Being asked to participate in setting their own goals and recommendations—even being spoken to as if they are customers rather than supplicants—could erode patient trust in the medical authority of their physician. There was some evidence from interviews with patients supporting this assessment. Several lay respondents said that they were unnerved by the style of younger physicians who asked patients what they want to do. Rather than feeling empowered, these respondents were left with the sense that their providers did not know what they were doing, or that it did not matter what approach was chosen.

Many providers cautioned that the best approach depends on the patient, and often patients simply prefer the old paternal style:

> In Japan, there are still quite a lot of people who like their doctor to order them, "Do this." I think the majority of older patients feel this way. And then fairly young people—people in their twenties, for example, and people who are fairly intelligent—have recently been looking up things on the Internet and coming in wanting to take a particular treatment approach or with questions about the efficacy of a particular medication. And then there are plenty of others who are just the opposite and have absolutely no idea about anything, so they want their doctor to make the decision for them.[9] (Endocrinologist, private hospital)

Like the American providers, Japanese providers argued that "some patients want to be told what to do." They assessed which patients would respond to orders and which would respond to cheerleading, which patients wanted to be given strict instructions and which wanted to participate in discussions with their provider about the best course of action. In a single morning, the same physician engaged with one patient according to the handbook protocols and the next with the gruffness stereotypical of the previous generation.

Deviation from polite discourse and the handbook version of respect for patients did not necessarily mean gruffness. Often, using informal language and speaking to patients in "short" registers was a way for clinicians to establish or acknowledge rapport with patients. Long inpatient stays, for example, fostered a familiar relationship between nurse and patient. One ward nurse explained during rounds that while they will start out using formal Japanese and family names with patients (and potentially their families as well), with time and necessity they moved to a first-name basis and more casual communication style. This sometimes meant referring to patients as -chan (a suffix usually reserved for children and young subordinates, but indicating a friendly relationship), speaking to them in simple short form, and using the regional dialect. The nurse explained that these techniques helped foster communication between nurse and patient, who sometimes only responded to simple, non-polite form Japanese. Keigo (respectful language) in particular may be hard for them to understand—or as the nurse put it, "pretty Japanese might be hard to understand." Using short form and the local Okayama dialect was easier on the patient, more comfortable, and more natural in tone.

Much like their American counterparts, Japanese physicians told the story of a shift from paternal to patient-centered medical practice. But where American providers focused on the responsibility of patients in their descriptions of patient-centered medicine, Japanese providers focused on respect for patients.

Medical Authority in the New Japan

Japanese providers approached their own medical authority as a tool for achieving results, relying on the high social status of biomedicine and play-acting at old-fashioned paternalistic medical practice when they believed it would be therapeutically effective. While they believed in building a Japanese medical community that has moved beyond "hierarchical relationships" between providers and patients in theory, like U.S.-based health care providers they were results-oriented when it came to their actual practices in the exam room. If behaving like a service industry employee according to handbook rules got results, they were satisfied—but when it did not, most shifted to other approaches. Japanese providers were as ecumenical in their approaches to patient interactions as their American counterparts.

Also much like American health care providers, Japanese physicians used medicalization as a tool to encourage positive patient behaviors. Physicians used the same "exercise prescription" strategy, for example, to make lifestyle recommendations seem more serious or concrete to their patients:

Basically, I calculate based on the amount of physical exercise. I calculate their METs (metabolic equivalent) and give them an exercise prescription. What is an exercise prescription? It's when you write a prescription for exercise. So having concretely calculated what is needed, I tell them specifically to do so much and to reduce calories so much. But really, even though I give it to the patient like that, the recommendations are extremely broad.[10] (Internist, private hospital)

This is the same approach used by the American endocrinologist quoted earlier, if a bit more numerically demanding. Writing prescriptions for otherwise abstract lifestyle changes both makes them more concrete and lends an air of medical authority. Tracking adherence to lifestyle change, like a medical intervention, gives it gravity and facilitates patients' faith that it will work.

This mix of patient-centered targets with the gravitas of medical authority to achieve better glycemic control with behavior change has made its way into formal intervention designs as well. Combining patient-centeredness with high external accountability, one recent intervention allowed patients to set their own goals apart from their providers, but then evaluated them on these goals at each visit (Yamamoto, Moyama, & Yano 2017). This approach was associated with sustainable improvements in glycemic control and decreased reliance on oral medication over two years.

In general, Japanese physicians also expressed tolerance for patients' use of alternative medicines, including Chinese medicine, supplements purchased online, massage, moxibustion, and religious practices—so long as they were able to check ingredients on any consumable medicines. Their greatest concerns revolved around the production of supplements and Chinese medicines in China, where the risk of contamination is perceived to be high. Japanese providers were less harsh on this point than their American counterparts. In interviews, they almost universally regarded the growth of health information on the Internet as a positive development. A female internist with a large number of type 2 diabetes patients explained that in many ways the Internet improved public awareness of type 2 diabetes:

All of my patients [with diabetes] know a lot about it [by the time I explain it]. In particular, the Internet has raised consciousness of the disease. There are people on the Internet who know a lot about diabetes, and people who don't know anything—that's a trend everywhere, I think. But for doctors as well as regular people, researching on the Internet can help us understand a lot.[11] (Internist, private hospital)

While recognizing that not all of the information available to patients on the Internet is accurate, this physician trusted her patients to discern. Further, she saw the Internet as a tool for primary care professionals, some of whom do not have as much experience treating patients with type 2 diabetes as she does. Patients and professionals alike should study the diabetes epidemic in whatever way they can, she argued, and the Internet makes that easier:

> A lot of people study privately. Anybody can do that on the Internet whenever they want. This is an era where people, especially young people, can do practically anything on their cell phones.[12] (Internist, private hospital)

With 100 million users in a country of only 127 million people, the use of technologically advanced smartphones in Japan has been widespread for decades (Tabuchi 2009). During the early fieldwork for this book, most were long, rectangular, clamshell-shaped devices with large screens used to access the Internet during long commutes. By the end, most younger adults had upgraded to conventional smartphones. In the early 2000s, approximately 71 percent of Japanese Internet users reported that they accessed the Internet with their cellular phone (Ministry of Public Management 2004, 2005).

Great Expectations and the Meaning of Care

Moving away from paternalism has not meant that Japanese medical practice more closely resembles American practice. Notably, Japanese physicians still ask for a level of discipline from patients that is relatively unusual in the United States. In contrast to American practitioners' low expectations of their type 2 diabetes patients, the Japanese physicians typically embraced high expectations of all their patients.

The difference in expectations about patient ability and the very possibility of controlling type 2 diabetes could lead to very different advice in the exam room. While American physicians reported relying on the simplest possible diet advice and encouraging patients to make miniscule changes to their daily lives, Japanese physicians asked their patients to make bold, time-consuming changes. A well-regarded endocrinologist at one of the most prestigious medical centers in the region described his approach to working with newly diagnosed type 2 diabetes patients:

> Ah, well. I promote the dietary approach to treatment more than the exercise approach. I'd say that it's about 85 percent diet . . . but, of

course, it's hard. Even though we say, "Okay, let's do this," it's hard for them to stick to it for me. Um, what I do a lot is tell people to weigh themselves four times per day and record the result. Then graph the results and look at them. Then the patient can think about how it makes them feel. For your own health, self-management — self-control — if you don't have that kind of program then I think it's hard. So I just ask them to please set themselves to a particular body weight. We look at their body weight, see how it measures up, and see how to improve it . . . Well, that I entrust to the patient.[13] (Endocrinologist, national medical center)

In many ways this is similar advice to what health care providers in the United States sample reported. But this endocrinologist's assumption that asking patients to weigh themselves four times a day and to actually graph the results is reasonable stands in sharp contrast to American practitioners' ideas about the limitations of their patients.

Many physicians asked patients with type 2 diabetes to keep small notebooks for tracking nutritional intake and, if necessary, use of oral medications, blood glucose readings, HbA1c values, and insulin use. Called *jiko kanri noto* (self-management notebooks), the booklets contained empty grids to guide patients in calculating their caloric intake and physical activity throughout the day. Patients brought the booklets to appointments, giving the physician a better sense of how well the patient managed his or her own lifestyle.

The reliance on patient discipline and general high expectations of patient participation — or at least cooperation — was common across the Japanese health care system. While physicians and other hospital staff complained in interviews that patients leave too much up to their physicians and thus use medical services for frivolous things, the basic expectations of patients are high. The private hospital's approach to medical records demonstrated this. All patient records were kept as electronic medical records, called an electronic carte, but individual patients were also issued a small, passport-sized booklet called a mini-carte. This booklet contains summaries of all their medical records and hospital visits, outpatient or inpatient. After each visit, an entry was pasted in by hand, and the patient brought the record home. If they visited another clinic or hospital or found themselves in an emergency medical situation, they could immediately present their health records to the new hospital.

According to the reception desk staff who checked in all outpatients and checked to make sure they had their necessary documents, patients took good care of their mini-cartes, rarely lost them, and generally remembered to bring them to every appointment — patients treated the carte as "precious" (*taisetsu no mono*). Indeed, over the course of three mornings, during which I observed more than 600 outpatients being processed, I only witnessed one patient who had forgotten her carte. In contrast, patients routinely forgot their insurance cards.

The mini-carte system is unusual in Japan and was not used at most of the other institutions I visited. It is so time-consuming for the nurses who must help prepare the summaries that it is inconceivable that the system could be used at the busier urban welfare hospital. But the fact that the suburban hospital successfully implemented the system and that the overwhelming majority of outpatients manage to bring their mini-carte to every visit was telling. Expectations of the general outpatient population were high, and these expectations were more or less met by the majority of regular patients.

The population of patients who continually fell short of expectations was easy to identify: unmarried men living alone. Providers noted privately that these patients' "loose" personalities mean that they never settled down with a wife to take care of them and that they probably enjoyed alcohol too frequently. While physicians, social workers, and nurses treated them with the utmost respect in interactions, in private they acknowledged among themselves that these irresponsible personalities probably could not be expected to properly manage a chronic condition like diabetes. Social workers were almost always enlisted to organize care for older, unmarried men.

But without the rhetoric of "choosing to be healthy" embraced by their American counterparts, Japanese physicians took a more active role in bringing their "loose" patients up to speed. Where the American providers emphasized patient responsibility, Japanese providers emphasized their own responsibility for managing patients' disease. Sometimes this active role led them to take actions that would be nearly unthinkable in an American context, like admitting a patient not in immediate physiological danger to the hospital because he was considered too undisciplined to successfully manage his diabetes. In other cases, the differences were subtler. Patients judged less capable of discipline were scheduled for appointments more frequently, sent to meet with the clinical social worker, and even weighed more often. (Normally *saishin* patients at the suburban hospital were trusted to self-report their own body weight when they arrive for exams, since they are expected to check for themselves frequently. This trust was not extended to those patients judged to have demonstrated self-management problems.) Thus, higher expectations of patients in general led directly to more intensive attention to those patients who did not meet the expectations surrounding self-management.

The development of a capacity for discipline and self-management was considered more critical for long-term success than simply being prescribed oral or injectable medication. Thus in exam room interactions, physicians and nurses emphasized the "eating treatment" for type 2 diabetes above the use of oral medication or injected insulin. While they acknowledged in interviews and conversations that this approach demanded much more of the patient, they pointed out that it was also much easier on the patient's body to enact difficult lifestyle changes than to simply treat to failure with medication. Nurse Kurokawa, a diabetes clinic nurse with twenty-five years of experience, explained:

> Medicine only . . . If you look at patients who are able to take oral medication, we tell them they can't just rely on the medicine. Eating is first and fundamental. They take medicine and they think, "Ah, now I'm ok." They feel relieved [and it is a bad thing].[14] (Outpatient clinic nurse, private suburban hospital)

It is best, then, to hold off on any kind of medication as long as possible. This encourages patients to work on their eating habits, which are the real key to managing type 2 diabetes over the long term. Otherwise, they may let their guard down.

Still, Japanese providers pointed out in interviews that lifestyle change is not easy. Like the American providers interviewed, Japanese physicians said that the hardest thing to explain to patients is that they will have to work to control their blood sugar for the rest of their lives:

> There are, of course, difficult cases where I need to keep explaining things. There are patients who have been admitted to the hospital and think that if they do their best for a short time they're cured. But that's not so. A disease is a disease, but this is a condition. So if the patient improves their eating and exercise habits, their blood glucose seems to drop easily. But it will rise just as easily as soon as they eat sweets. Telling them that [just because their blood sugar is under control] doesn't mean that their disease is cured . . . I explain it, but I really wonder if it gets through to them.[15] (Diabetes-specialized endocrinologist, national medical center/university medical center)

Like the providers interviewed in the United States, Japanese physicians recognized type 2 diabetes to be a particularly, peculiarly difficult diagnosis.

Patients in both countries expected to be able to take a pill and be cured, or work hard at lifestyle change for a while and be done. But there is no diabetes cure, only diabetes management. And diabetes management requires permanent, radical lifestyle change for most patients—a prospect that is no easier for Japanese patients than it is for their counterparts in the United States.

However, Japanese providers used much more positive language to describe the possibility of controlling diabetes than American providers. Diabetes was characterized as "85 percent diet" and the parameters of managing the condition could be "calculated" for patients. Self-management was "entrusted" to patients and their families, who were praised for "doing their best" and characterized as capable. When they did not prove so capable, physicians actively attempted to control the condition on their behalf, though in ways that would seem intrusive in an American context.

Japanese patients are not intrinsically more disciplined than American patients. But their efforts to understand and manage their disease take place in a setting that may support lifestyle change more consistently. The level of discipline Japanese providers expected of their patients was easier to support and, in some cases, to enforce than in the United States thanks to a much higher frequency of patient contact. For example, when asked how patients reacted to initial diagnoses of type 2 diabetes, the Japanese physicians pointed out that most of their patients knew that the diagnosis was coming for five years or more. Free, annual physicals provided for in Japanese law and required of workers for most large companies mean that most patients know from an early point that they are progressing toward type 2 diabetes. By the time most patients are diagnosed with type 2 diabetes, the word "diabetes" is familiar. And once they are diagnosed, they can expect to be seen by a physician several times a year. In contrast, American providers estimated that the average type 2 diabetes patient in the United States lived with the condition for approximately seven years before finally being diagnosed.

Further, admitting patients for the sake of education or preparation like Dr. Saito did for Ichiro is not unusual in Japan. Usually, patients are admitted not because they have misbehaved in some way, but because it is thought to be the best way to train them to perform the tasks associated with managing their diabetes. At the urban welfare hospital, a small ward was set up just for patients learning to administer insulin or, less commonly, home dialysis. Patients were admitted and supervised for five days when they first began using insulin. In contrast, most patients at American medical centers receive less than an hour of outpatient instruction before they are sent home with insulin.

Frequency of patient contact and the occasional hospital stay are important for vulnerable populations because the severity of type 2 diabetes is not usually evident to patients until it is too late. Diabetes develops over months and years with no pain or obvious symptoms before resulting in serious complications. As more than one nurse put it, diabetes simply "doesn't hurt enough." Patients require professional attention not only for an accurate diagnosis but also for a reasonably accurate assessment of the disease's progression. The Japanese physicians, like the U.S.-based health care providers, were pragmatic in their approach to relationships with patients. Because they were results-oriented rather than dogmatic, most physicians embraced the ideal of patient-centered medicine in interviews, hospital meetings, and formal encounters, only to behave in very different ways in the exam room. The same doctor changed his or her style of addressing and treating patients from patient to patient, sometimes in the span of only a few minutes. Similarly, physicians self-consciously medicalized the idea of lifestyle change when they thought that lending lifestyle change the weight of their own medical authority would motivate the patient.

Japanese physicians, in interviews as well as in their actual interactions with patients in exam rooms, evidenced a greater degree of trust and higher expectations of their patients than American providers. They were more optimistic about the possibility of controlling diabetes over the long term and about patients' chances at good health. This seemingly small difference led to major differences in the exam room, from physicians' preference for dietary intervention over medication to the justification of what might otherwise seem to be patronizing treatment of "undisciplined" patients.

Professional Strategies Across Cultures

Despite differences, health care providers in the United States and Japan approach encounters with patients in a number of remarkably similar ways. Practitioners in both countries took a pragmatic approach to negotiating with patients. Practitioners in both countries recognized the power of medicalizing lifestyle recommendations when they explained treatment options to patients, self-consciously relying on medical authority to "sell" behavioral changes to some patients. These chapters, then, are partially about similarity—that despite major institutional differences and patient mixes, health care providers in the United States and Japan employ a similar spectrum of strategies.

But there was one difference between exam room strategies that emerged with important consequences for management of the type 2 diabetes epidemic in each country: expectations. While American providers were fatalistic and even pessimistic about the possibility of controlling diabetes, Japanese providers were relatively optimistic. While American health care providers in the sample reported self-consciously monitoring and depressing their expectations of patients, Japanese providers embraced expectations of their patients that seemed almost unreasonably high. One might think that Japanese physicians would give their patients a break, since unlike the majority of U.S.-based respondents, the majority of Japan-based physicians in this study reported that they either had type 2 diabetes themselves, had impaired glucose tolerance, or were worried about getting type 2 diabetes. But Japanese physicians consistently evidenced higher expectations of their patients in interviews and in practice, with consequences for patient care.

The Japanese physicians may have risked overestimating their patients, but they rarely risked underestimating them. American providers protected their patients from the psychological risks associated with attempting bold lifestyle changes, but they risked affirming patient assumptions that real change is impossible and that their condition is not within their control. The difference for providers may have been little more than a subtly different attitude, but the consequences of provider expectations for patients could be great.

CHAPTER SIX

Diabetes at Home

Explanatory Models in Everyday Practice

In chapter 3, I argued that the diabetes epidemic in Japan is cast as a morality tale about the nature of Japanese identity, emphasizing the particularity of diabetes risk to the Japanese body in contemporary Japan. But this narrative emerged when respondents were asked about the diabetes *epidemic*, not their personal experience with type 2 diabetes. When asked instead about daily preventative practices, personal worries, and causal theories to explain their own illness or the illness of someone close to them, participants instead articulated explanatory models centered on the disruption of healthy, ordered rhythms. When the level is shifted from the population to the personal, explanations shift as well.

When discussing personal health philosophies and explanations of their own health and illness, Japanese interview participants first associated health with having an order or rhythm to one's life. Observing regular, unchanging hours for core activities like waking, eating, and bathing were identified as key to a healthy life. Type 2 diabetes patients in the sample articulated a similar causal understanding of the relationship between living an ordered life and maintaining health as other respondents. Or, rather, patients pointed to a relationship between living or having lived an "unordered" life and the onset of their illness.

But the responsibility for this temporal maintenance falls largely on women: women work to organize loved ones' time into a healthy, regular rhythm. Gender played an even clearer role in the illness experiences of type 2 diabetes patients and their families. Male patients described worry over their condition but offered few causal narratives. The wives, daughters, and sisters of male patients, however, often offered explanatory models on behalf of their loved one. Women worked not only to manage diabetes on behalf of loved ones but to give it meaning.

Finally, the majority of Japanese physicians I interviewed said that they personally worried about developing type 2 diabetes. This stands in sharp contrast to the American providers, only one of whom expressed concern. Most of the Japanese physicians reported a sense of inadequacy at reducing their personal risk of diabetes and other types of illness by living an "ordered" life, which they felt was out of the question given their professional obligations. The American providers, on the other hand, felt invulnerable to diabetes because of their privilege and access to healthful things.

Private Experiences of Health and Illness in Japan

Illness narratives draw our attention to the interface between agency and social structure. These narratives are simultaneously strategic tools with which patients restructure social roles and articulations of how their lives are shaped by political-economic forces beyond their control (Mendenhall et al. 2010). Narrative is an autonomous act to make sense of and to renegotiate one's social roles. Yet illness narratives often implicate the social, political, and economic forces outside the patient's power. Moreover, narratives are built, at least in part, from local materials. Cancer patients, for example, construct causal stories about their illnesses using "local moral constructs framed within distinct cultural and social perspectives" (Hunt 1998, 2000, cited in Mendenhall et al. 2010).

When asked to talk about the nature of health, laypeople and providers alike emphasized imposing order and regulation on the body as a general route to wellness. Patients with a diagnosis, members of the general public who worried about getting diabetes, and people who expressed no worry about facing chronic disease themselves mostly agreed on one thing: the ordered life can maintain health, while the disordered life leads to illness.

This section will first discuss the model of the ordered life that respondents associated with health and then the narratives about disorder type 2 diabetes patients offered when asked why they thought they developed type 2 diabetes. Finally, the discussion will turn to the particular private experiences of Japanese physicians, who experience higher rates of type 2 diabetes than their American counterparts and were more likely to report personal worries about the disease.

The Ordered Life and Classification of Time

When asked, "In general, what is the best way to stay healthy?" most lay respondents described an "ordered" life, or a life according to rules. These respondents described the ordered life in one of two ways. The most common responses were *"kisoku tadashii seikatsu"* or *"kisokutekina seikatsu,"* phrases with only minor differences in meaning. The former, literally "rule—correct—lifestyle," suggests orderly or clocklike. The latter, literally "rule-like lifestyle," is closer to regular or regulated. For the purposes of this chapter, I will treat them as synonymous in meaning and translate them both to mean orderly. The remainder of respondents provided concrete descriptions or examples of healthy lifestyles that accorded with this emphasis on regulation, explicit rules, an organization of time, such as by emphasizing that activities like eating and sleeping must take place at set times.

The connection between the descriptor "orderly" and set times was made explicitly by several respondents, so I treat responses referring to the importance of set times for certain activities as belonging in the same category as those that explicitly identify an orderly life with health. For example, one 24-year-old urban office worker who considered herself a basically healthy person and was not worried about suffering from type 2 diabetes in the future defined a healthy life as an orderly life, and an orderly life as one in which daily activities take place at set times according to a rhythm.

> INTERVIEWER: What sort of lifestyle do you think best prevents you from getting sick?
> MARIKO: An orderly life. Yes.
> INTERVIEWER: What does that mean concretely?
> MARIKO: Waking up every morning at a set time, eating breakfast at a set time, consuming food with balanced nutrition, and keeping an orderly rhythm to one's life.[1]

When respondents described an orderly life, what they typically meant was a life where one is able to keep regular hours and perform daily activities at set, unchanging times with few surprises. The ability to observe temporal boundaries was key to health maintenance for most respondents, and this is part of what is expressed in the phrases *kisokutadashii* and *kisokuteki na seikatsu*. The work of maintaining health is at least in part the work of maintaining appropriate boundaries.

Mary Douglas argued that the erection of such boundaries is a creative, ordering act engaged in through one form or another in all human societies (Douglas 1966). In Douglas's reading, dirt and disorder are symbolically synonymous. "In chasing dirt," she writes, "in papering, decorating, tidying, we are not governed by anxiety to escape disease, but are positively reordering our environment. There is nothing fearful or unreasoning in our dirt-avoidance: it is a creative moment, an attempt to relate form to function, to make unity of experience" (Douglas 1966: 3). The construction and observation of symbolic boundaries is a creative expression of order.

A central premise of this book is that these creative expressions of order, in the form of explanatory models—sets of interrelated assumptions about the basic nature of health and illness—reference symbolic structures, which may vary across cultural context. Medical anthropologists of Japan—Japanese as well as non-Japanese—have devoted much work to theorizing about the underlying symbolic structure of Japanese health attitudes (see Lock 1980, 1995; Traphagan 2004; Yoro 1996; Namihira 2005). Ohnuki-Tierney's work on the underlying symbolic structure of Japanese health behaviors and attitudes also emphasizes the centrality of boundary-making. She argues that the underlying symbolic structure of health beliefs in Japan is characterized by attention to boundaries between inside and outside, insider and outsider, based on characteristically Japanese spatial classifications. The inside is by its nature clean in a spiritual sense, the outside is dirty. In Ohnuki-Tierney's usage, "outside" (*soto*) does not refer to natural, "unpeopled" spaces. Rather, the outside is peopled with outsiders, strangers, those who do not belong to the household (*ie*): "people-dirt" (Ohnuki-Tierney 1984).

The spaces that delineate inside from outside require constant policing and care. In the traditional Japanese home, the *genkan* delineates this boundary; it is the space through which one passes to reach the inner spaces of the home, where one removes shoes carrying the dirt and germs of the outside. Boundary-making spaces are fraught with the uncertainty of being neither inside nor outside, neither completely dirty nor completely clean in a symbolic sense. They are vulnerable spaces, spaces that carry the risk of contamination and miscegenation. This renders boundaries ontologically dangerous spaces. The boundary between inside and outside is the place where one is most vulnerable to contamination. Thus the *genkan* must be the site of symbolic cleansing and shedding, the mouth must be protected from breathing in dirty air by masks, and uncertain periods between seasons are considered the time when one is most vulnerable to illness (Ohnuki-Tierney 1984).

Symbolic boundary-making may be rooted in Japanese spatial classification, but as the final example suggests, such boundaries could easily extend to temporal classification. The in-depth interviews collected here, though, suggest that the classification of time is central to understandings of wellness. Charmaz (1991) observes that patients' classification of time affects whether or not their experience of chronic illness is integrated into their sense of self or experienced as merely an interruption, a way-station between previous health and future health (Charmaz 1991: 23, 30). How individuals and communities define and experience time can have profound consequences for patient identities, determining (among other things) whether or not the self is put on hold by illness experience or is altered and grown by illness.

The relationship between appropriate, ordered organization of time and health does not exist only in general or abstract discussions of health, illness, and prevention. The role of time boundaries also emerged in discussions of prevention of and specific risk factors for type 2 diabetes, demonstrating that the temporal classification and its underlying symbolic structure directly influence the ways that respondents imagine and actually address risk for type 2 diabetes. For example, respondents identified "night eating" as a risk factor for type 2 diabetes. Eating at night, later than a reasonable dinnertime, was thought to be more dangerous to one's health than eating at other times. The night eating behavior they described is distinct from night eating syndrome (NES), a disturbed eating pattern associated with high calorie intake (Striegel-Moore et al. 2008). Rather than late-night snacking, these respondents described dinner out of place as the primary problem. Evidence from a recent cohort study, in fact, supports this supposition, finding that late-night dinner patterns were independently associated with poor glycemic control among people living with type 2 diabetes (Sakai et al. 2018). The respondents discussed here anticipated this study by more than five years.

The head nurse at the suburban hospital worried informally about the tendency toward night eating she saw among hospital physicians. She warned me several times not to lapse into the doctors' bad habits just because I shared an office with them. In an interview several months after we began working together, she explained that night eating was part of the larger problem of an unordered lifestyle.

> That and not living an ordered life [is the reason for rising rates of diabetes].[2] You can't be unregulated, can you? Do you understand what *fukisoku* (unordered/ unregulated) means? In a word, it's . . . um . . . it's like not eating in proper fashion in the morning, noon, and night, but just eating in the morning and at night. Hmm, how to put it? It's not eating at set times. Or letting it get really late, and eating late at night. I think there is a connection between that sort of chaotic eating [and diabetes]. Yes. [Nods head emphatically.][3] (Head nurse, suburban private hospital)

This nurse applied the concept of temporal disorganization directly to risk for type 2 diabetes. What is "chaotic" about the type of eating she singled out is not high calorie content or poor nutrition, but rather eating out of order. The risk of the eating originates in its inappropriate timing, not its content. Thus the policing of time boundaries is a central theme in the management of the body, both in abstract conceptions and in the specific case of diabetes.

Eating is hardly the only daily activity that must take place at set, appropriate times. A sixty-three-year-old housewife in the rural sample, for example, defined a properly ordered life as being most obviously about regulated eating, but cautioned that going to bed early and waking up earlier were also important components. She felt that restraining oneself from the temptation to nap during daytime hours and waking up at a set (preferably early) time each morning were critical. The ordered life necessarily included set times not only for eating, but also for sleeping and bathing. It is the adherence to a rhythmic, regular organization of one's time that renders a lifestyle ordered rather than its content.

Of course, saying that the ordered life protects from disaster and actually living according to the sort of temporal organization respondents identified as ideal are two different things entirely. The difference between articulating an ideal pattern of behavior and applying it to one's own life creates tension, especially for respondents who have lived with chronic illness. Life is inherently arrhythmic. Unexpected stressors appear at work, a cold snap makes physical activity suddenly less appealing, a child or grandchild gets sick. Or one is merely tired from the long work hours and commutes that are commonplace in Japan, and forcing oneself to keep a clocklike schedule gradually becomes exhausting, until the effort is abandoned altogether.

The difference between normative assessments of healthy behavior and actual practice was never more evident than in conversations between family members. Families live together, eat together, and care about one another enough to notice when loved ones are not keeping to the rules they believe can keep them healthy. Women especially commented that they worried for fathers or husbands, who knew that they ought to eat or sleep better but did not. Family members are close enough, both socially and physically, to call one another out when words and behavior do not match.

Family members in the rural sample frequently called one another out in the middle of actual interviews. In Hosekijima, the town from which rural respondents were drawn, interviews typically took place in homes with traditional open floor plans. Family members passed in and out, occasionally commenting on the conversation. In some cases, married couples asked to be interviewed together (something that never happened among urban dwellers). When family members were interviewed together or simply present in the house during an interview, they often chided one another about the difference between words and practice.

One such interview with a sixty-two-year-old parking lot security guard called Daisuke took place in an old but beautifully kept farmhouse near the family's rice paddies in Hosekijima. The house had several wide rooms with tatami flooring, divided by thin sliding wood panels, all of which were thrown open or taken off their tracks to allow air to circulate on a sultry July day. Daisuke's sister-in-law, Akiko, an active woman in her late sixties who made her living farming rice with her husband, passed in and out bringing chilled noodles and tea for us. Each time she would linger to comment, ask questions, encourage her brother-in-law to show off his prized collection of *daruma* figures or sing me a traditional song, fuss with the fan, or simply tease one or both of us.[4]

When Daisuke mentioned that he never got colds or other minor illnesses, I wanted to know his secret. I asked "Since you said you never get colds, what do you think is the best way to protect one's health?" He paused a moment to think, then responded,

DAISUKE: An orderly lifestyle, sleep, relaxation, and nutrition.
INTERVIEWER: You sound like a public notice.
AKIKO: Even though he says that, he doesn't keep to it!
DAISUKE: They say, "Sleep well and eat nutritiously."
AKIKO: What he says and what he does are not equal. But I suppose everyone is like that.[5]

Daisuke lived in an idyllic-seeming farmhouse in a rural area, but there were few jobs in Hosekijima and the family's rice cultivation was too small scale to support everyone. He commuted nearly an hour to his job as a parking lot security guard in the city, where he worked irregular hours and sometimes took night shifts. Akiko worried over him and his irregular schedule constantly. "He never married," she told me on another occasion. "So I worry about him."

Typically it was women who engage in talking, teasing, or wheedling family members into a more ordered life. In Japan, where women have a much lower rate of participation in the formal labor force, particularly during peak childbearing years (Ogasawara 1998), women shoulder most of the responsibility for domestic work. This means that women—as wives, mothers, sisters, or daughters caring for aging parents—often feel that they bear the responsibility for enforcing the correct temporal organization on their families in the name of health and well-being.

I don't think I really told [my children and husband] with words, but I woke them up at the same time every day, made sure they got protein in proper fashion in the morning, gave them vitamins, things like that. I told them they had to eat carbohydrates and tried to make them eat properly. And at night after dinner is over we don't eat anything . . . . I told them to go to bed early. I guess that's about all I was careful about. Other than that, there wasn't really anything. It's because I'm sort of loose. I brought them up in a loose way.[6] (Homemaker, rural Japan)

It is notable that this seventy-two-year-old woman, now a grandmother, considered the way she raised her children to be "loose," a word with negative connotations in Japan suggesting a kind of irresponsible leniency. Enforcing regular hours in the day and an appropriate eating pattern of protein in the morning and carbohydrates during the day seemed to her to be the least she could do for her family.

The idea that enforcing a *kisoku tadashii* rhythm was a feminine task was widespread. In the previous chapter, I observed that physicians and co-medicals focused on men with a "loose" lifestyle as being at the highest risk for uncontrolled diabetes. What put these men as risk was not so much their love of sake and "stand-up" ramen—food products beloved by most stereotypical salarymen—but the lack of women in their lives to help regulate their time and behavior. When Dr. Saito hospitalized Ichiro, she was influenced by the consideration that he had no wife or daughter to guide his behavior. If Ichiro had had a wife, the wife almost certainly would have been enlisted to help, and Dr. Saito would have been less likely to admit him. Without women regulating their lives, the ordered life is much harder for men like Ichiro to attain.

The Experience of Illness

In this section, I examine the relationship between the conceptualization of well-being and temporal classification through the narratives of three patients with type 2 diabetes: Kimiko, Tomoko, and Rei. Kimiko had lived with a diabetes diagnosis for more than ten years. Tomoko was first diagnosed with type 2 diabetes in the time between our first and second interviews. Rei identified as having "borderline" type 2 diabetes, and says she lives in expectation of crossing the imaginary line into what she calls "exact diabetes."

Kimiko: A Decade with Diabetes

When Kimiko, a fifty-seven-year-old graduate of the hospital's diabetes education program and regular visitor to the outpatient clinic, was asked why she thought she of all people got diabetes, she responded decisively, "An unordered life. Unregulated eating." Pressed for more details, she explained:

> I was irregular in my habits. [I worked at the] barber shop. It was always, "Please just wait five minutes." When a customer came in I would go immediately. I would just slurp up my miso at meals because I might have to rush to my job at any time. If you say five minutes and the customer waits seven minutes, they are just hideous . . . So I would just postpone adjusting [my lifestyle]. I couldn't rest like I ought to have because I was busy. Now I have more free time, though.[7] (Retiree and diabetes education class graduate, suburban private hospital)

Kimiko echoed other laypeople's evaluation of diabetes risk and general risk for illness, not just in her evaluation of her previous lifestyle as unordered (*fukisoku*) but also in her particular emphasis on the issue of time. Her job did not allow her to observe boundaries around periods of time. She could not have a time designated for eating and a time designated for working that could be kept day after day. The lines between different categories of time were muddied, and she did (or could do) nothing to make them clear. She located the source of her own condition not just in failing to control her calorie consumption, but in her inability to control the *temporal conditions under which she consumed*.

When Kimiko described postponing adjusting her lifestyle to something healthier, she said *"zuruzuru,"* a mimetic word that connotes both the sound made when slurping noodles and the act of postponing or procrastinating. The mindless slurping of noodles and the thoughtless postponing of a more regular, ordered life are parallel acts in her description. When she described the factors that contributed to her diabetes, she emphasized the lack of intentionality in her former lifestyle. Her life with a diabetes diagnosis, though, was radically different. She retired from full-time work cutting hair, is seen by Dr. Saito once or twice a month, and attends diabetes education classes at the suburban hospital at least once a week. Her life is now ordered by a schedule of meals chosen intentionally for their nutritional content, frequent visits to the hospital for appointments or classes, daily walks, and other activities that express her new commitment to herself and her own health.

In Kimiko's narrative, chronic illness occasioned self-discovery—and justified self-care. In her old life, her time was organized by the whims of other people, for the benefit of other people. Diabetes gave Kimiko not only occasion to examine the temporal organization of her life but also the justification for focusing more on herself and her own well-being. In Kimiko's telling, her life with type 2 diabetes is more rhythmic and more fulfilling than the life that she feels caused her type 2 diabetes. Her illness narrative is a resource that allowed her to restructure her social roles and exercise agency.

Tomoko: Two Weeks Down, a Lifetime to Go

Tomoko was a tall, slim woman in her midfifties. She lived in a rural area but was well traveled and cosmopolitan in her tastes. The café she owned served largely Italian fare, and she brightened when she described her adventurous youth, when she traveled around the world and fell in love with a Tibetan cowboy. Though we spoke in Japanese, I knew that she had a gift for languages and spoke English well. She told me that she finds Japan stifling after too much time spent at home; it is only when she travels abroad that she feels able to breathe and really look at people. And her every-other-year trips are more than just spiritually restorative—she explained forcefully that when she sees the doctor after being abroad for several weeks, he tells her that her blood pressure has dropped and her cholesterol has improved.

The first time I interviewed Tomoko was at her café in Hosekijima. She flitted back and forth between her customers, considering my odd questions as she cooked pasta and toasted bread with cheese to order. At this first meeting, Tomoko was not worried about type 2 diabetes. She told me she had high cholesterol, which she attributed to her love of Italian food and cheese, but said, "But there isn't any real relationship between diabetes and cholesterol, right?" When I told her that high cholesterol is generally considered to be a risk factor for type 2 diabetes, she was surprised. At that first meeting, she told me that the healthiest life is just a "regular, well-ordered lifestyle," adding ironically that "not eating too much delicious food" probably helped as well.[8]

Our second meeting was nearly a year later. After chatting over the course of a leisurely walk on her day off, we found a shop specializing in fresh tofu that could serve a calorie-controlled meal. She had been diagnosed with type 2 diabetes two weeks before and scrutinized the two set meals available at the shop trying to determine which would be better for her. "I'm learning now," she explained.

When I asked her how she discovered she has type 2 diabetes, she returned to cholesterol. "From the beginning," she explained, "I had high cholesterol." She had known about her cholesterol for more than five years and described how she was diagnosed, even recounting her conversation with the doctor. At our first meeting, Tomoko did not believe there was any connection between cholesterol and diabetes, but now she linked the two conditions.

One day in the year between our two interviews, Tomoko went to donate blood with a mutual friend. When they took her blood they told her that she should have blood work done to check for type 2 diabetes. She was surprised, and put off going to her physician for the test for months. She even went to the clinic for her cholesterol medication without mentioning that she had heard she should be tested for diabetes. Because she was a small business owner and did not work for a large company, there were no rules requiring annual physicals or diabetes screenings.

But then one day she cut her foot. When she went to the doctor, she finally mentioned the blood test. Her physician tested her immediately and told her she had type 2 diabetes. "I had never thought of diabetes before that," she said.[9] After her initial shock came fear:

> By the time I first heard, the doctor said it was already not so good. For me, my diabetes didn't have a start. It was already pretty bad. So I thought, "Ahh!" I thought about horrible things like losing my vision or not being able to walk on my trips abroad.[10]

Tomoko, still reeling from her initial diagnosis, experienced her illness as acute rather than chronic. Since she was diagnosed with full-blown type 2 diabetes, rather than easing into her illness with a progression from at-risk to prediabetes to diabetes, her diabetes was an unwelcome interruption. And rather than enabling her to further develop her sense of self as Kimiko said her diabetes allowed her to do, Tomoko's diabetes threatens the aspects of her identity she holds most dear: her ability to work independently and her ability to go on adventures abroad.

When directly asked why she thought she developed type 2 diabetes, Tomoko responded:

> Of course, I think the number one reason is my DNA. DNA plus . . . what else? My eating and stress. For a long time, my lifestyle has not been very good. That's what I've been thinking about the most.[11]

Like many respondents, Tomoko first listed a genetic predisposition, which she tied to Japanese identity in other parts of the interview, as an explanation for her illness. But she quickly added other factors that she dwells on more than the genetic explanation: her unhealthy lifestyle. When pressed about what aspects of her lifestyle were not good, Tomoko returned again to the stress brought on by living in Japanese society, her unordered work and eating schedule as a small business owner, and her disordered sleep schedule. After having suffered from insomnia for years, she believed that an irregular and unsatisfying sleep schedule must have contributed to her illness. And her disordered eating, the result of both a hectic work schedule at the restaurant and personal struggles with eating and body image, was probably another reason for her current condition.

When describing the etiology of her illness, Tomoko did not focus on a specific event as many populations in the United States do (Poss & Jezewski 2002; Schoenberg et al. 2005). Rather, she depicted her illness as the result of a combination of genetic risk, stress, and chronic disorder in her schedule. Unlike Kimiko, her narrative does not liberate her.

Rei: Life on the Borderline

Rei was sixty-six and lived in the city, where she took classes at a downtown library in her free time. She approached me after I presented my research at one of the library's free classes, introducing herself as a "borderline diabetic." Rei rattled off her statistics as soon as we sat down to chat in the library's international exchange center. "My hemoglobin is 6.0 or 6.1 right now, but I want to lower it to around 5.8," she said, almost before we had exchanged greetings. "I was diagnosed five years ago, but the lowest I've gotten it is 5.9."

Rei approached her prediabetes like a baseball player, keeping track of her record highs and lows, calculating her personal best and average HbA1c levels. (Results of the HbA1c test indicate average blood glucose over up to three months; they are a simple measure of overall diabetes control.)

> Yes, well, I can't exactly say that I have diabetes right now, but if I'm
> not careful I'll become diabetic. So I'm careful about food and exercise.
> I was told to be. And since I didn't want to end up diabetic I really
> applied myself. And right now I am completely diabetes-free. I've been
> told that for my age, restraining my hemoglobin to 6.0 or under is pretty
> good. I was young, but I'm already turning sixty-six.[12]

Rei seemed to actually take pleasure in monitoring her lab test results. She thought of them as scores and used them to monitor the grace with which she was aging. She even compared her results to friends, family, and neighbors to assess how well she is doing relative to those around her.

Rei thought of diabetes as a threat to which she was responding with the same level of care and competence with which she ran her household and shepherded her overachieving children through school. Her constant self-monitoring revolved around one overarching goal: do not pass over the hash mark that denotes "diabetic."

> Being told I have diabetes—that would be awful. When you're told that, there are severe restrictions on your food. Just that alone would be really hard, and so I don't want to be told I have diabetes. I don't want to be told I have diabetes, and so I am controlling myself.[13]

Even though her quest to avoid full-blown diabetes led her to place restrictions on her diet, she did not imagine them to be restrictions in the same way they would be if she crossed the line into diabetic territory. Rei saw her current nutritional planning and caloric restriction as "controlling myself." If she were to cross the line into type 2 diabetes, however, the diet restrictions would control her.

These three women offered different, highly personal illness narratives and explanatory models for their illness, but all three emphasized the relationship between temporal organization and well-being. Kimiko's causal narrative connected her inability to organize her own time according to a regular, healthy rhythm to the onset of diabetes. Tomoko located the source of her diabetes in her irregular, stressful life as the owner of a small restaurant. Rei was barely interested in the cause of her diabetes at all but used her prediabetes to organize her self-identity and as a lens through which to understand natural, healthy aging.

Gender and Illness Experience

Something else stands out about the patients mentioned above: they are all women. While many female type 2 diabetes patients articulated illness narratives, men were more reticent and more likely to offer stock responses. It is possible—even likely—that the fact that their interviewer was a woman contributed to their reticence. But in other interactions, male colleagues, even those who became friends or with whom I had daily contact, spoke little of their own experience of chronic illness. Despite the fact that a significant proportion of the physicians at the private hospital said in interviews that they had either been diagnosed with type 2 diabetes or thought that they were on the road to diabetes, male physicians never brought illness up with one another in social interactions. Silences can be as important as rich narratives. That the men with type 2 diabetes or prediabetes did not seem as eager to talk about their experience of diabetes does not necessarily mean that they had not considered it as actively as the women, but it does suggest that their illness occupies a different place in their sense of self.

The fact that the primary method of prevention and management that laypeople and patients broached in interviews was the organization of time and the exercise of intentionality in domestic activities cannot be overlooked. The preparation of food, the timing of meals, and even making time for exercise and recreation are clearly gendered. This is evidenced not only by physicians' worry over men with diabetes who lack a wife or daughter to take care of them but by men's reactions to diabetes diagnoses. One physician, for example, pointed out that he knew he should eat better and exercise more, but his stay-at-home wife was in charge of meals and he did not have time for exercise. "Playing tennis is the sort of thing my wife does during the day," he said. Not only cooking, but recreational sports and exercise seemed like feminine activities to some older Japanese men.

The division of household labor places women in charge of health and well-being for their families. As such, many female respondents expressed illness narratives on behalf of men in their lives. In other words, the women who performed both the domestic labor (in the form of cooking and organizing time) and the emotional labor (in the form of worrying and ascribing meaning) on behalf of men in their life were more eager to narrativize the illness than men in the sample. Just as women organized time and meals on behalf of the men in their lives, they also articulated illness narratives on behalf of those men.

While men are usually at slightly higher risk for type 2 diabetes than women, worry over the illness in Japan is feminized. Indeed, fear of type 2 diabetes and its complications is surprisingly widespread among middle-aged and older women. Of fifty-three women surveyed at a women-only gym in Hosekijima, 68 percent said they worried regularly about type 2 diabetes. The women who said they were afraid of getting diabetes were asked to write down their personal reason for worrying. They were not given preformed categories. Of those who were worried, eleven cited a family connection to diabetes in their written response. Ten said they like to eat or liked to eat sweet things, and that they worried this would put them at risk. Seven described the disease and its complications, calling it "scary" or "incurable." One in this category simply wrote, "Because at my workplace I see many people who have diabetes."[14] Still another wrote, "Because it is a sickness that is with you until death."[15] In categories of their own, one woman said that she had heard that soon one in every three or four people could have diabetes, and another said that she was worried about diabetes because it was something that happened alongside growing old, and she would soon grow old. The remaining six provided no answer.

The women were also asked for their thoughts on the best way to avoid diabetes. The phrasing of the question, "In order to try to avoid diabetes, what do you think is good to do?" could be interpreted as a leading question; respondents were never asked whether or not it was possible to avoid diabetes.[16] However, the phrasing in Japanese is open enough to allow for the common set phrase "There is nothing to be done" (*Shikata ga nai*). Still, no one responded that there was nothing to be done. Responses ran the familiar spectrum of balanced eating habits, exercise, an ordered lifestyle, and a correct, upright life.

Perhaps more interesting were the responses of those who said they were *not* worried about type 2 diabetes. More than half of the respondents in this group did not write a response to the question about their personal reasons for *not* being worried, but the ones who did emphasized their own management. One respondent wrote, "[I am not worried] because I am managing myself and getting medical checkups (*kenshin*)."[17] Another wrote, "Because I'm making an effort not to eat too many sweet things."[18] Five of the eight respondents in this category said that they monitored themselves through frequent doctor visits, so there was no need to worry. "I have blood work done once a month. I think there is nothing abnormal about my blood glucose."[19] Only one cited a lack of family history as a reason for their lack of worry. Rather, they pointed to their own monitoring or the monitoring of their doctor.

The Doctor with Diabetes

In sharp contrast to the health care providers interviewed in the United States, the majority of physicians interviewed in Japan reported that they themselves had type 2 diabetes, prediabetes, or thought they were otherwise at high risk for developing type 2 diabetes. A little over half of the Japanese physicians interviewed cited a personal connection to type 2 diabetes. In contrast, only one of the twenty diabetes health care providers interviewed in the United States said they ever felt concerned about getting type 2 diabetes themselves.

In the United States, nearly half of all physicians are Caucasian (Bureau of Labor Statistics 2010). All other things being equal, those of European descent are thought to be at lower risk for type 2 diabetes than those of African, Asian, or American indigenous descent (Glumer et al. 2006). Further, U.S.-based primary care physicians enjoy high socioeconomic status and a median income of $189,044 (Bureau of Labor Statistics 2010). (And physicians in medical specialties have an annual median income of more than $330,000.) The Bureau of Labor Statistics does not collect income data for nurse practitioners, but CNN reported that the median annual income for nurse practitioners is around $85,000 (2009). In the United States, high socioeconomic position across the life course is negatively correlated with risk for type 2 diabetes (Maty et al. 2010). The overrepresentation of people of European descent among practicing physicians and their high average income both place U.S.-based physicians at lower social risk for type 2 diabetes than most of their patients.

In Japan, however, physicians may actually be at a slightly higher risk for type 2 diabetes than the rest of the population. There is no reason to believe that the distribution of genetic risk for type 2 diabetes varies between doctors and patients in Japan, but doctors are more likely to work long, irregular hours. Patients' and providers' models of diabetes in both the United States and Japan closely associate stress with the development of insulin resistance, and it would not be surprising if Japanese physicians actually suffer from type 2 diabetes at a *higher* rate than the rest of the population. Regardless, these physicians self-identified as a population at higher than average risk.

Thus, even those medical professionals who do not think they are at risk because of genetic predisposition worried that their hectic, stressful lifestyle put them at elevated risk of developing diabetes. Long shifts with unpredictable work made it difficult to live an ordered life or maintain control over their own time. Like the patient who worked at a barbershop and had to abandon plans to serve customers, physicians in Japan live at the mercy of their pagers and mobile phones. Even relatively senior physicians spend uncomfortably long periods "on call" and are required to do service to the hospital with occasional night shifts. At the suburban private hospital even the vice president, a cardiologist, was on call every weekend.

Physicians treated the prospect of their own chronic illness with a touch of dark humor and a sense of inevitability. When asked if he ever worried about getting type 2 diabetes himself, a young, visibly fit diabetologist at the prestigious national medical center paused for a moment, then answered,

Ah, well. I have a family history. A lot of them have diabetes, so I think I probably will get it. [laughter][20] (Diabetologist, national medical center)

Dr. Hatasa refrained from musing about how his work affects his expectation of growing ill himself, but rather reflected on how his expectation of becoming ill eventually affects the way he interacts with patients. He explained that knowing he would someday be a type 2 diabetes patient himself made him a more engaged, energetic health care provider.

Other physicians who worked closely with type 2 diabetes patients described it as a consciousness-raising experience. Another diabetologist at the national medical center said that she worried about type 2 diabetes even though she didn't think she necessarily faced a genetic risk:

If I am not self-conscious about my own daily life habits, the amount of fat or oil in my diet, for example, then it gradually grows [out of control]. The amount of sugar I consume too. The fact that a regular Pocari Sweat drink, for example—sports drinks or stuff you drink from PET bottles—is loaded with sugar is something I didn't even know until I became a doctor myself. So I guess nobody really realizes it. Since I'm conscious of this now, as much as possible . . . in the old days I really liked snacking, but now I try as much as possible not to eat snacks. I've tried to reduce oily foods as much as possible too. I just don't like exercise very much and can't keep it up, but at work I try to use the stairs [rather than the elevator] as much as I can. But even keeping that up all the time can be difficult. Every once in a while I resolve again to make a real effort to be careful. "Let's be careful," I remind myself.[21] (Diabetologist, national medical center)

This physician's sense of her own risk grew directly from her experience educating and counseling type 2 diabetes patients. Patient interaction inspired self-reflection. American providers, in contrast, said that their experiences treating diabetes did not precipitate concerns about their own personal health or the health of their families.

Most of the time, when physicians were asked whether or not they themselves worried about diabetes, they interpreted the question as one about prevention and the daily rhythm of their own lives. Even physicians not worried about diabetes expressed a sense of the inadequacy of their own preventative measures, of their inability to enact the lifestyle they believe could ensure health for themselves and their families. While they daily asked for discipline and control from their type 2 diabetes patients, the physicians who did not worry about the condition for themselves were aware that they did not practice the same discipline and control in their own lives. Dr. Furukawa, an internist at the national medical center, explained:

> INTERVIEWER: Are you worried about diabetes for your own family?
> DR. FURUKAWA: Not so much for my family. We make an effort to have well-regulated (*kisoku tadashii*) food, balanced meals, but nothing in particular . . . Well, it's not limited to diabetes. We think of whole body health. But it's not perfect. Even though we make an effort, it's not perfect. That's my sense of it.[22]

In fact, this type of response was very similar to the attitude evinced by most American providers. A generic emphasis on regulation, moderation, and balance guided provider responses to questions about their own personal or family health in both countries.

Conclusions

Lay respondents with no personal history of diabetes articulated an understanding of health maintenance that revolved around the idea of an ordered life. Order was thought to come from careful adherence to a classification of time that associated certain times with certain activities and erected boundaries between them. Having a "rhythm" to one's life and observing regular, unchanging hours for core activities like waking, eating, and bathing were identified as key to a healthy life. But the responsibility for this temporal maintenance fell to women, who worked to organize their loved ones' time into a healthy, regular rhythm. Men without female family members were thus thought to be particularly at risk of illness. Type 2 diabetes patients articulated a similar model. Most patients offered causal stories related to an unordered lifestyle. But diabetes patients' relationship to time was more complex than that of laypeople. For some, the illness became a source of new order in their present lives.

The gendering of the domestic and emotional labor surrounding illness was even more evident in interviews with patients than with laypeople. Female patients were more talkative about their illness in interviews and more likely to tell their illness as a story, complete with narrative arc. Male patients described worry over their condition but offered few causal narratives. The wives, daughters, and sisters of male patients, however, offered explanatory models and illness narratives *on behalf* of their loved one.

When asked to talk about the nature of health, Japanese laypeople and health care providers alike emphasized imposing order and regulation on the body as a general route to wellness. Patients with a type 2 diabetes diagnosis, members of the general public who worried about getting diabetes or some other lifestyle disease, and people who expressed no worry about facing chronic disease all provided a similar rationale whether prompted by questions about type 2 diabetes or basic healthy lifestyles: the ordered life can maintain health, while the disordered life leads to illness.

Conclusion

Diabetes and Its Discontents

Nearly eight years after I first began research for this book, I sat uncomfortably in another room with institutional floors, balancing a bound medical register on my lap. Around me, patients held handkerchiefs or surgical masks over their mouths and leaned against the wall or into plastic chairs. A community health worker sat nearby with a new patient, asking him how many people slept under the same roof in his home and carefully recording his answers. She would need them to initiate contact investigation for tuberculosis, an infectious disease that now kills more people than HIV and malaria combined.

At public-sector clinics like this one in Kampala, Uganda, newly diagnosed tuberculosis patients are recorded in paper registers. They are tested for HIV, initiated on treatment for tuberculosis, and then followed on paper for at least six months of pills and follow-up tests. Despite this, a quarter of these Ugandan patients will experience treatment failure. Although tuberculosis is curable, 16 percent will be dead within the year.

I was scanning the register for a key piece of information about each patient that might help identify which among them were most likely to experience treatment failure or death as a result of tuberculosis: their fasting blood glucose level. Each time I reached a patient with significantly elevated random or fasting blood glucose suggestive of diabetes, I added a tick in my notebook and tried to find any record of treatment for diabetes. Only two of the six clinics I had visited that week had metformin on hand, though. Even when patients are initiated on treatment for diabetes, many do not continue because essential medicines for diabetes are not consistently available.

The face of global diabetes is changing dramatically. An astounding 80 percent of diabetes cases now occur in low- and middle-income countries (Critchley et al. 2017). Low-income countries like Uganda face rising rates of type 2 diabetes, even as their health systems remain focused on battling epidemics of microbial diseases like tuberculosis and HIV/AIDS. Among rapidly developing middle-income countries, China and India alone are home to 110 million and 69 million diabetes patients, respectively. Much as the social epidemiology of type 2 diabetes shifted in the United States from high-income to low-income populations, its geopolitical epidemiology is shifting fast. By 2015, the United States had dropped to forty-second place in International Diabetes Federation diabetes prevalence rankings.

In its global travels beyond high-income nations, diabetes carries some familiar baggage: the burden of stigma, and the perennial challenge of managing a chronic disease when face-to-face time with skilled health care providers is a precious commodity. This baggage is transformed by its new contexts, though. In Uganda, for example, fat stigma is rare; fatness is socially valued and strongly associated with health, strength, and beauty. The weight *loss* associated with diabetes progression is more likely to have negative social consequences in a setting where changes to body mass are associated with HIV.

AS NIKOLAS ROSE has written in his critique of its overuse and undertheorization, "The term medicalization might be the starting point of an analysis, a sign of a need for an analysis, but it should not be the conclusion of an analysis" (2007b: 701). In the preceding pages, I began from the observation that processes associated with (bio)medicalization are underway in Japan as in the United States. As the very nature of well-being is reoriented around biomedicine, both the pathways to and practices of biomedical care become more diverse and more complex. Providers' recommendations become socially "subjective, collaborative, and highly uncertain" (Spencer 2018: 5).

Biomedicalization does not flatten out differences so much as it proliferates them. As the biomedical paradigm has become central to lay systems of meaning, the language and ideas of biomedicine are imbued with cultural meanings (Rose 2007a). In this way, medicine can shape and reorganize cultural meanings on a grand scale. But the reverse also occurs: the cultural meanings that arise from lay systems shape the patient-provider encounters that lie at the heart of the practice of medicine. These meetings of lay and medical systems of meaning are sense-making events in which patients and providers practice culture, and biomedicines and lay cultures co-produce one another.

In the preceding chapters, I considered how and why evidence-based practice varies. The providers I described all acted in the best interests of their patients, on the basis of shared evidence, and with reference to increasingly global standards. They reached clinical decisions and communicated them to patients. But to do that, they relied on local knowledge and on narratives about diabetes constructed, in part, from local materials. In the two different settings, they formed different assessments of their patients' cognitive and psychosocial resources, reached different conclusions about patients' capacity for change, and defined their own duty to ensure change in different terms. They tailored their clinical decision-making—about dietary recommendations, oral medication, or self-management—in ways that reflected these different ways of thinking. In this way, local knowledge and localized interactions with patients shaped the ways in which physicians interpreted and enacted global standards and best practices.

Even as consensus around evidence has globalized in biomedicine, then, distinct patterns of practice persist in these two biomedical communities. These patterns of practice relate, in part, to the different resources providers and patients draw on to imagine how and why diabetes affects their communities. In chapter 1, I set out three guiding questions to explore how cultural resources from different settings enable different narratives to become pervasive, and how these narratives might ultimately contribute to different practices. These questions are not meant to be explanatory devices. Rather, they provide a framework for thinking about the practice of culture in medical encounters in the context of intensifying biomedicalization.

What are appropriate and healthy uses of the body? I argued that the dominant narrative in the United States framed healthy uses of the body as those that are "natural." The natural is imagined to be universal to all people. The reverse of natural, *un*healthy uses are those identified with stress and modernity, like "scary chemicals" in food and the temptations of convenience. In Japan, the dominant narrative framed healthy uses of the body as those that are "traditional." Traditional ways of treating the body included consuming foods such as rice and fish or traveling on foot. This dominant narrative emphasized the particularity of Japanese practices to Japan, rhetorically linking the well-being of Japanese bodies and Japanese culture. When used as a resource to explain or communicate about diabetes, this narrative subtly oriented medical encounters for diabetes around the performance of Japanese identity.

Who exercises legitimate medical authority, and how? In both the United States and Japan, medical authority is demonstrated through membership in a privileged professional community, but it is imprinted by setting-specific racial, gender, and generational inequalities. Thus, while health care providers in both countries stress that their authority comes from membership in a professional community with access to specialized knowledge unavailable to laypeople, in practice their authority is buttressed or eroded by the systems of power, authority, and legitimacy that permeate their respective settings. In the increasingly unequal United States, status differences between provider and patient were often profound, and providers voiced frustration over the foreign social universe of non-middle-class patients. In Japan, income differences between provider and patient (and across patients) were less stark, but expectations about the gender (masculine) and generation (graying) of the most trusted practitioners permeated medical encounters. Further, the character and extent of medical authority differ—Japanese physicians were able and willing to make extraordinary demands of their patients. American physicians hesitated to cross a line, privileging patient autonomy and distancing themselves from autonomous choices that they judged poor.

If health is a responsibility, whose responsibility is it? U.S.-based providers focused on the individual as the unit at which health and illness occurred, and the unit that was ultimately responsible for maintaining health. Japanese providers, patients, and other lay people, on the other hand, asserted the individual, the family, the health care system, and the nation itself as key sites of health and illness. The patient's (female) family and health care provider took partial responsibility for health maintenance and the management of chronic illness.

Thus, in the United States, biomedicalization and a capitalist ethic of productivity and individual responsibility are mutually reinforcing: the individual is continually reinscribed as the primary category of being and the object of medicine. In Japan, biomedicalization intertwines with discourses of nationhood, membership in a purportedly unique racial-cultural community, and gendered domestic labor. The cases described here suggest that while biomedicalization does not flatten, its targets are reshaped in legible ways by its contexts. As biomedicalization renders interactions between providers and patients more uncertain and more collaborative, the cultural resources that they bring to those encounters become more—not less—relevant. In an era of biomedicalization, then, the character of biomedicine is continually shaped and reshaped by the tools its participants bring, reinforcing and reinscribing local assumptions in medical encounters.

Methodological Appendix

In this appendix, I describe my methodological orientation and debts, the practical methods used to collect the data used in this book, and the data itself. I conclude with a section noting my own place in the communities that took me in, taught me, and offered up professional and personal experiences for this project.

Methodology

This project is an inductive, qualitative, comparative study of the plurality of biomedicine (Kleinman 1995) that used an inductive "grounded theory" approach to producing and interpreting sociological knowledge from interview data. In grounded theory, data collection tools are continually reevaluated and redeveloped throughout the collection process (Charmaz 1983, 1990, 1991; Glaser & Strauss 1967; Lofland & Lofland 1984; Strauss 1987). As a comparative, case-based study, it relied on data from a variety of sources, including themes and categories emerging from these interviews, to generate a clearer understanding of the relationship between biomedicalization, globalization, biomedical practice, and context.

Grounded theory can mean many things. There are three major approaches to grounded theory to choose from, not to mention a variety of alternative approaches (Miller & Salkind 2002). Even among the three best-recognized approaches, there remain significant differences in epistemological commitment and assessment of methodological rigor. Of these three, the most rigid approach embraces a systematic design, with prescribed data analysis steps that include open coding, axial coding, selective coding, and finally the production of an explicit, visual representation of the theory generated (Strauss & Corbin 1990; Miller & Salkind 2002). The more flexible emerging design formed as a critique of this rigid procedural approach. Glaser (1992) emphasizes that the point of grounded theory is to allow categories to emerge from the data, rather than to rely on preconceived categories and constantly submit to rigid procedures. A third and final approach, constructivist design, rejects clearly delineated analytical stages, diagrams that "obscure" experience, and overdetermined theoretical constructs (Charmaz 1990, 2000; Miller & Salkind 2002).

My approach was closest to that of Charmaz (2000) or Lamont (2000), but combines elements of all three of these variants. Though the size and linguistic complexity of my data led me to rely on a methodical approach toward organizing and analyzing, including open and axial coding along the lines of Strauss and Corbin (1990) for the first 143 interviews, I believe that the flexible, interpretive approach of Charmaz (1990, 1991, 2000) is more sensitive to the subjective experience of participants. To the extent possible in a project with a single researcher for hundreds of participants sharing their ideas in two languages, I attempted to emulate Charmaz's close attention to the subjective meanings shared by participants and rejection of obscure language and theoretical constructs (Charmaz 1990; Miller & Salkind 2002). I subscribe to the claim that a good analysis and ensuing theory will "fit the realities in the eyes of participants, practitioners, and researchers" (Miller & Salkind 2002).

Methods

Before beginning the interview process in the Japanese field sites, I interacted with health care providers, patients, and the laypeople I interviewed in unstructured encounters outside the context of the interview, which many participants in Japan treated as a formal occasion. I shared offices with physicians and shadowed them on their rounds and clinic hours for several months. I sat in nurses' stations and chatted over lunch. I attempted (unsuccessfully) to make myself useful at the reception desk of a busy suburban hospital, and wore a sash as a greeter in waiting rooms, giving directions to patients seeking a particular clinic or ward. I participated in diabetes education classes and clinical examinations, seeing the same patients week after week until we were fixtures in one another's schedules. I had the point system and the financial organization of the Japanese health care system explained to me countless times by medical administrators and senior physicians gravely concerned about the future of Japan's unique health system.

Participation in and observation of the "natural discourse" of physicians and patients was especially important because interviews alone are less constrained by the realities of actually working with patients. They thus allow physicians and other biomedical professionals to talk about medical practice in a "more abstract or idealized fashion" (Loewe & Freeman 2000). In this project, interviews were "time-out" moments where physicians and patients could present idealized depictions of the patient-provider relationship and their own models of diabetes. Participant observation, on the other hand, could offer insight into the lived experience of clinic life. Combining participant observation with interviews allowed me to compare discourses in the formal setting of the interview with more natural discourses in the exam room, classroom, and waiting room.

I carried out semistructured interviews with members of each population using an interview instrument designed to elicit discussion not only of one's own experience treating or living with illness, but also one's perception of how and why others became sick. A central question I put to participants in this project was "Why is there an epidemic of type 2 diabetes at all?" The interview instrument was not static; as I conducted more interviews (and sometimes interviewed the same individual on multiple occasions), I returned to and adjusted the interview guide. Semistructured interviews were treated as an iterative process, in which the interview instrument was adjusted to accommodate ideas and categories that emerged in previous interviews.

I returned to the instrument at regular intervals to add questions and prompts that touched on emerging themes I had not anticipated at the time the instrument was created. In line with classic grounded theory approaches, I reevaluated the instrument after approximately every ten new interviews. This process was repeated through 115 initial interviews in Japan, and 28 in the United States. The subsequent interviews in

Japan were carried out with a structured interview guide that did not change. While the U.S. sample was much smaller, it was still within the range grounded theory methodologists consider adequate, and I approached those interviews with the same openness to new themes. By the end of my interviews with U.S.-based providers, the cadence and themes of these interviews had become familiar, indicating that I had reached saturation.

There was reason to believe that respondents in the rural sample from Hosekijima may have very different explanatory models, health practices, idioms, and concerns from the urban/suburban sample. Rural Japan is demographically and socioeconomically distinct from urban Japan—it is grayer, more agricultural, and has lower average incomes (Traphagan 2004). Health maintenance attitudes and practices may differ between urban and rural communities (Traphagan 2004; Lock 1980). Therefore, I used a pre-interview survey instrument to examine potential differences in responses regarding health beliefs before beginning interviews in Hosekijima. In fact, the broad contours of the responses to questions about prevention were very similar across the rural and urban samples.

After transcribing the digitally recorded interviews, I coded and analyzed responses in three stages. Two of the stages were similar to the open coding and axial coding steps embraced by Strauss and Corbin (1990) discussed above. In the open coding step, I built a "codebook" by reviewing the transcripts line by line and tagging repeated themes, equivalencies, or connections between ideas that emerged from the interviewees themselves. In the second stage, I carried out a second line-by-line check using the whole (at this stage, unwieldy) codebook in order to code sections that were incompletely coded in the first stage because some themes had not yet been assigned codes. In the third stage, I applied axial coding to identify references to complex concepts such as "risk is universal/particular," "Western food does not match Japanese bodies," and "biomedical etiology." I applied axial codes using automated search-and-code features rather than line by line. Although I characterize this step as axial coding, I did not approach the process as rigidly as Strauss and Corbin (1990). Instead, I thought of it as a highly methodical version of Charmaz's (1990) more flexible strategy for collecting and analyzing interview data.

After coding was complete, I drew verbatim statements on the themes that had emerged as relevant from the dataset through simple searches for codes and code co-occurrence. This produced pages of quotes for every thematic subsection. From those pages, I chose quotes that represented the others and touched on core themes. Before quotes were used in chapters, I examined them again in the context of the interview.

In the case of the Japanese verbatim statements, I translated the statements to English myself with reference to the overall context of the interview. I endeavored to present the Japanese statements in language that did justice to their complexity and, in many cases, banality. Any errors are entirely my own. Translating quotes can introduce awkwardness into the statement that was not present in its original language. Whenever I translated a statement, I include the original Japanese transcript in an endnote, so that readers of Japanese can have access to the original wording.

Data

The Hosekijima sample was recruited using a modified snowball sample, relying on multiple close ties to the community developed over a period of several years. The sample is entirely composed of laypeople; there are no physicians or nurses, though there are many people professionally involved in care for the elderly. One family of rice farmers provided introductions to at least thirty other families in the northern, agricultural half of the community. I spent many days biking around the more rural parts of the town with the family's energetic matriarch, who joked that I was a "replacement daughter" (*ko no kawari*) standing in for one of her own children who had gone abroad. Keiko and her family made it their mission to introduce me to the people who made up their social world, and many of those individuals and the individuals they referred are included in the sample. Other Hosekijima participants were recruited through two public school teachers, a foreign language teacher, and the owner of a small restaurant. Further participants were recruited in turn from the individuals they introduced.

The urban sample was composed of respondents living and working within the boundaries of Okayama City, a prefectural capital of more than 650,000 people. Okayama City is the twentieth largest city in Japan and became a national "designated city" during the course of my fieldwork. Though it is urban by American standards, Japanese from other parts of Japan as well as Okayama itself refer to Okayama City derisively as *inaka*—countryside. Okayama City has a pattern of urban density similar to post–World War II American cities. It is urban in the city center and suburban in the outlying communities that have been absorbed into the city in the past two decades.

I recruited the city sample using a snowball approach beginning from multiple initial contacts. I did not conduct any interviews in either location until I had completed approximately five months of near-daily participant observation in a variety of medical settings, which meant that by the time I began interviews I was integrated into the city's medical community. Professional contacts from my field sites at a suburban private hospital, an urban public welfare hospital, an urban university medical center, and a suburban *kampo* (Chinese medicine) clinic were my first urban interview participants. They in turn introduced me to colleagues at other health care sites and recommended me to patients and friends.

Nonprofessionals were more difficult to access in the urban environment. I relied on personal contacts including fellow graduate students, a city librarian, a professor, and two friends working as youth organizers for the prefecture—"youth" in this case means people ranging in age from 19 to 35—to introduce me into social networks outside the direct patient population for the hospitals at which I worked. I also presented five- to ten-minute explanations of my research to adult education classes at an urban library once a month and invited participants to contact me. The librarians kept my business cards and short descriptions of my research on their reference desk and scheduled interviews for me when patrons expressed interest in participating.

The interviews are only part of the diverse collection of evidence I draw on for this project. I also reference eleven months of fieldwork in several medical facilities in western Japan, including six months of participant observation in the outpatient diabetes clinic of a suburban private hospital, a month at an urban welfare hospital, repeated visits to a *kampo* clinic, and a week spent shadowing house calls with a "country doctor" in a rural part of the prefecture.[1] During this time I was permitted to sit in on interactions between doctors, nurses, and patients in exam rooms and spent hundreds of hours observing and participating in the daily operation of the clinics. I also participated in two diabetes education programs: one run like a support group that incorporated friendly, accessible explanations of type 2 diabetes and its management, and the other a more formal, classroom-style program. Part of my responsibility (and privilege) as a visiting member of the hospital staff was to attend weekly all-hospital assemblies, doctors' administrative meetings, and a variety of social events with medical colleagues throughout the year.[2]

In addition to the interviews and ethnographic component, I distributed a short pre-interview instrument to members of an all-women gym in Hosekijima. The 53 participants responded to open format questions about preventative medicine and ideas about how to stay healthy. I informally focus-grouped the Japanese instrument with several informants in Hosekijima: a worker at an eldercare facility, a rice farmer, a housewife, and two teachers. They argued for several changes in wording and organization, most of which were incorporated into the final instrument.

The purpose of the pre-interview instrument was to determine the best approach to semistructured interviews in the rural context rather than to provide the basis for a quantitative analysis, but the results are nonetheless interesting and are mentioned in some of the preceding chapters. Because the instrument was set out on the front desk of the gym and it is impossible to determine how many potential respondents saw the survey but did not fill it out, it is impossible to calculate a response rate. The gym is part of a franchise in which membership to any location entitles members to use the facilities at any other location. However the manager estimates that the Hosekijima location attracts approximately 100 regular members each week for near-daily low-impact workouts and camaraderie.

To validate findings from the initial 115 interviews collected in Okayama, I collaborated with research assistants and students from the School of Political Science and Economics at Meiji University to collect a further 216 semistructured interviews from 80 families as part of the Japan Multigenerational Interview project (J-MIP). The J-MIP protocol combined basic sociodemographic information that can be matched to items in the Japan General Social Survey (JGSS) with a semistructured interview covering health beliefs, health practices, and health care experiences related to noncommunicable diseases including diabetes. These interviews were coded in Dedoose, a web 2.0 tool for mixed-methods analysis that allows codes to be applied directly to digital audio.

The empirical component for my second research location, North Carolina, is much smaller. I gathered 28 in-depth, semistructured interviews from medical professionals and lay respondents in Durham, North Carolina. Because an enormous body of work already exists on the explanatory models of American type 2 diabetes patients, I did not collect interview data from type 2 diabetes patients and instead reference several large-N studies using similar semistructured interview techniques (Loewe & Freeman 2000; Schoenberg et al. 2005; Lange & Piette 2006; Borovoy & Hine 2008; Chesla et al. 2000, 2009; Mann et al. 2009; McSweeney et al. 1997).

I recruited medical professionals working with type 2 diabetes patients at various local medical centers through an endocrinology fellow working in the Duke University Medical Center, who generously contacted colleagues on my behalf. Initial interviews led to further introductions. Medical professionals in my North Carolina sample work in a variety of contexts, from major university medical centers to a regional hospital to a neighborhood clinic to the local VA hospital. They came from a variety of professional backgrounds; the sample included endocrinologists, internists, nurse practitioners, physicians' assistants, a nursing professor, nurses, and diabetes educators. Lay participants were recruited either through a snowball sample or through posters placed at various locations around Durham.

The U.S.-based empirical component of this project was on a much smaller scale than the Japan-based work. This lopsided approach is premised on the presence of a large, high-quality body of work on the sociology of health in the United States. Priority was given to establishing an empirical foundation for comparing Japan and the United States, given that a great deal of thoughtful work in medical sociology and the sociology of health is already conducted in the United States. Because a reasonable amount of empirical evidence already existed for the U.S. case, I gave more attention to gathering evidence in Japan, which is relatively understudied.

The lopsided approach is also premised on my own training and cultural background. As a U.S.-trained, American sociologist, American cultural and institutional approaches to health and health care are far more familiar to me than those of Japan. When I conduct fieldwork or analyze data from Japan, the United States serves as an implicit reference point.

A Note on Being an Outsider

In Japan, and especially in the relatively rural prefecture where I conducted most fieldwork for this project, I am visibly marked as a foreigner and an outsider. While my first name looks misleadingly like a common Japanese name, my hair, eyes, and odd surname all mark me as different. Upon meeting in person, there was no mistaking me for a member of the Japanese ethnic or political community. My status as a foreigner living in Japan and speaking Japanese was remarked upon by participants and certainly affected all parts of the research process, from gaining permission to work at my clinical field sites, to interview recruitment, to how respondents described and discussed the diseases during interviews.

Further, Japanese medical establishments tend to be rigidly gendered spaces. Most physicians are men; nurses are women. Medical clerks may be either, but the hospital leadership at all the sites included in this project was entirely male. Nurses' stations were female spaces, occasionally visited by physicians and technicians with their own workspaces elsewhere. Shared physicians' offices were usually male spaces; except for one or two days a week when a part-time female internist visited the hospital, my cubicle was the only one of twenty in our shared office occupied by a woman. When nurses or female medical clerks came to our office for any reason they announced themselves as they entered, apologizing for interrupting. In contrast, neither physicians from other offices nor male administrators and clerks announced themselves as they entered or left.

In this male space, I was the only female. My placement in this office by the hospital president reflected a sort of ambiguity in my status that remained throughout my fieldwork. As a foreigner, a woman, a Ph.D. student from a university highly regarded by Japanese medical professionals and researchers, a sociologist, and later an assistant professor at a well-known Tokyo university, it was never clear where I was to fit in. The hospital president placed me in a prominent cubicle in the largest shared physicians' office and gave me a white coat, but also made my immediate supervisor the head nurse. As a result, I passed between the clearly delineated masculine and feminine spaces daily, standing behind the head nurse at morning all-hospital meetings but also attending the all-doctor meetings closed to nurses and other staff and spending the majority of my time shadowing male physicians.

In the shared office, I was the only female, the only foreigner, and the only non-physician. In the nursing stations, I was the only woman in a lab coat. In the hallways, I was the only non-Asian foreigner. When a delegation of volunteers visited from another hospital, my colleagues were introduced in a sentence. My introduction took an entire conversation.

This outsider status, and the resulting ambiguity about my place in the hospital hierarchy, was exactly what allowed me to enter any of these spaces at all. The confusion over how I fit into the overlapping hierarchies of gender, age, and profession contributed to a certain degree of privilege. My presence in the physicians' office scrambled so many gender boundaries that it was simply easier for most of my colleagues there to treat me as an honorary man. After the first flush of formality in the autumn, by midwinter I was invited to parties for medical staff and learned to decipher the peculiar informal speech patterns of middle-aged men, as colleagues gradually stopped speaking to me in more formal registers. I became worried that I was picking up the bad habits of "men's speech" myself. A generous speech-language pathologist took it upon herself to tutor me in more ladylike speech so I could avoid embarrassing myself.

After several months, I believe it was clear to everyone that I had *some* place at my primary hospital. I showed up three days a week for twelve-hour shifts, attended all major meetings, gave several presentations, interviewed many of the medical and nursing staff, and participated in social activities. I do not think it ever seemed clear to anyone, though, what exactly my place was or ought to be. Instead, the small hospital and its staff simply got used to having me around. Had I been Japanese myself or even appeared liminally Japanese, had I not presented such a jumble of status contradictions to the social world of the hospital, I doubt I would have been able to traverse so many of its social spaces.

Being an outsider can sometimes mean not knowing the right questions. I often asked the wrong questions during my fieldwork in both countries. But outsiderness also makes it easier to ask questions at all. My childish insistence on asking, "But *why?*" would likely not have been humored in a Japanese colleague or researcher. Instead, my irritating barrages of questions were not only humored but embraced and eventually even anticipated. Interviewees and hospital staff took on the role of teachers. As a foreigner I was assumed to be approximately on par with a small child when it came to understanding Japanese history and culture.

Age, too, marked me as different from the vast majority of colleagues, informants and interviewees involved in this research. The participating physicians at my primary field site tended to be older; many had children in my age range. This may have contributed to a certain tendency among my office mates to take care of me, to explain things that they assumed must be mysterious to me, and even to attempt to guide my research.

The president of the suburban hospital, for example, saw me in the narrow hallway behind the outpatient clinic one winter morning and approached me. "I realized that to understand the future of the Japanese health care system you must understand DPC. We don't use DPC here yet. I will send you to [the welfare hospital] for a few weeks to study DPC," he concluded. "Prepare yourself today." Within days all my previous commitments at the suburban hospital were canceled, I was put in front of the welfare hospital board to formally ask for permission to observe their medical center, and I found myself "studying abroad" at a large, urban welfare hospital. My relative lack of interest in DPC, a system for managing inpatients, was a nonissue to the well-meaning president. I did not return to regular shifts at the private hospital until a month later. On other occasions I was unexpectedly shipped off to a geriatric hospital, an elder day-care facility, and to shadow a country doctor making house calls, all because one of my superiors came to the conclusion that I simply had to see some other clinical setting in order to "understand Japanese medicine."

Spending a month "studying abroad" at the urban welfare hospital was, in fact, a valuable and elucidating experience. This project would have suffered without the relationships, interviews, and observations I had the privilege of forming there. I am very fortunate that the hospital president was thoughtful enough to secure the opportunity for me. But the point is that neither the plan nor the timing of my sojourn to the welfare hospital were my own. The president saw it as his responsibility to direct my education in the organization and practice of Japanese health care. Especially given my relative youth, this made perfect sense within the hierarchy of the hospital—he was the teacher, I was the student.

This student-teacher dynamic characterized many of my relationships with key informants, whether in Okayama medical establishments or over tea on tatami mats in Hosekijima farmhouses. Even once I became a professor, this dynamic persisted. I am, in fact, relieved that it has persisted. I continue to learn more from my colleagues and community in Okayama than I could ever hope to convey. Any insights contained in the preceding pages are theirs. Any errors, on the other hand, are certainly my own.

Notes

Introduction

1. Under the current system, all Japanese citizens receive medical insurance through one of several sources, depending on their employment situation. The most basic medical insurance covers 70 percent of medical and pharmaceutical costs, leaving a patient burden of 30 percent. The patient burden for those who receive health insurance from large corporate entities is often lower, around 20 percent. Meanwhile, health care costs are controlled by a point system set by the government; each visit, procedure, product, and prescription medicine is assigned a point value.

2. There are many ways to measure the relative efficiency of a health care system, but the most basic is to simply compare percentage of gross domestic product (GDP) spent on health care to measures of population health. Japan spends approximately 8 percent of its GDP on health care and enjoys some of the best scores for population health in the world (OECD 2006). According to OECD data, the United States spends twice as much as Japan on health care as a percentage of its GDP, but its infant mortality rate remains twice that of Japan. More dramatic social stratification, stratified health care access, and lifestyle factors in the United States probably contribute to this difference. Nonetheless, the wholesale creation of an inexpensive, accessible, top-notch health care system may be one of the most impressive and enduring successes of postwar Japan.

3. For an English language report, see "Japan, Seeking Trim Waists, Measures Millions," *New York Times*, June 13, 2008, http://www.nytimes.com/2008/06/13/world/asia/13fat.html.

4. See article above.

5. The 2012 Nobel Prize was awarded jointly to John Gurdon and Shinya Yamanaka.

6. To protect respondents' privacy, the name of the town has been changed.

Chapter One

1. Some of the most horrific crimes against humanity sponsored by the wartime government involved pseudomedical human experimentation. The infamous Unit 731 and associated units infected, assaulted, and vivisected thousands of men, women, and children to observe the progression of a variety of infectious diseases and traumatic injuries, including bubonic plague, smallpox, cholera, loss of limb, starvation, severe burns, and lethal exposure to radiation through x-rays. This large-scale lethal human experimentation was supposed to provide an empirical basis for Japan's biological warfare program, estimates for the lethality of weapons such as grenades at various ranges, and a better understanding of battle injuries. The ubiquity of grotesque

for the sake of grotesque, such as experiments where limbs were amputated and reattached to other parts or sides of the body, betrays the orgy of violence against colonial bodies (mostly Chinese) that drove the enterprise.

2. Japan's recent per capita pharmaceutical expenditure is above the OECD average, but significantly lower than the United States (OECD 2011). This is largely because Japan has been much more successful than the United States at reducing expenditures through price controls.

3. Comparative data on health consultations in OECD countries is available at http://stats.oecd.org/.

4. Japanese primetime television, famous for its wacky quiz shows, has even featured some medical quiz shows. In a recent iteration, medical interns from famous medical schools compete *Jeopardy*-style to identify a mystery disease based on a short vignette. Their answers are evaluated by a professor and senior physician and discussed by the requisite panel of minor television celebrities.

5. In Kleinman's original formulation, explanatory models are highly personal stories about how and why illness affects a particular person. I use the term "explanatory model" more broadly than many researchers do, because I assume that all people have explanatory models for illnesses with which they have any familiarity, even those with which they do not have personal or professional experience. Explanatory models are stories about why type 2 diabetes affects a particular person, but the explanatory model itself can be articulated by anyone—friends, family, health care providers, acquaintances, and even total strangers can have explanatory models about illness that are not their own.

Chapter Two

1. In one important exception, Rock (2003) examines the construction of type 2 diabetes as a major public health problem in Canadian public policy. Rock (2005) analyzes the presentation of type 2 diabetes in two Canadian newspapers and two American magazines, and is used throughout this discussion.

2. This possibility is raised in a recent and already influential popular book, *Diabetes Rising: How a Rare Disease Became a Modern Pandemic, and What to Do About It* by Dan Hurley.

3. For examples, see http://www.diabetesforums.com, http://www.diabetesdaily.com, and http://www.dlife.com.

4. For an example, see the archived thread "Did I Cause My Diabetes?" at http://www.diabetesforums.com/forum/type-2-diabetes/43416-did-i-cause-my.html (accessed May 2018). This discussion runs more than 150 posts long, and includes all the elements common to divisive discussion of who carries the blame for rising rates of type 2 diabetes: posters with type 1 diabetes who argue that nutrition and lifestyle are the primary etiologic factors, posters with type 2 diabetes who call those with type 1 diabetes self-righteous, serious questioning of the causal relationship between obesity and diabetes by those with type 2 diabetes, suspicion that toxic chemicals rather than calories are responsible for the epidemics of type 2 diabetes and obesity, and accusa-

tions that type 1 diabetes patients believe they are morally superior to type 2 diabetes patients.

5. For examples, see "Did I Cause My Diabetes?" cited above, or "What's Up with My Docs?" at http://www.diabetesforums.com/forum/type-2-diabetes/58365-whats -up-my-docs.html (accessed May 2018).

Chapter Three

1. The claim that Japan is environmentally unique also surfaces, when convenient. A Japanese trade minister anticipating the Nagano Olympics once famously claimed that Japanese snow was different from snow in the rest of the world, thus necessitating the use of Japan-made ski equipment. "Foreign skis will not work in Japan because Japanese snow is different," he argued in the midst of a protectionist trade dispute (Woodall 1997).

2. The debate over the place of Japanese children raised overseas captures this sense of uncertainty. As postwar Japan grew to be a major economic power, Japanese companies sent elite executives, managers, and workers to staff their locations overseas. Many of these men—and they were almost always men—brought families. Their children, born in Japan and raised overseas, seem credibly bicultural on the surface. They are fluent in multiple languages. Many were even sent back to Japan during their summer vacations in America or Europe in an attempt to ensure their continued linguistic and cultural development as Japanese. As the first generation of these overseas nationals have become adults, they have been the subject of a number of newspaper editorials in Japan on "the returnee child problem" (*kikokushijo mondai*) (Goodman 1992). The editorials typically argue that the overseas children possess critical skills in foreign language and culture that Japan needs to embrace in order to remain globally competitive. But the context of these articles is always that the overseas children are *not* embraced, that they are somehow *not* truly Japanese, and that there is something just a little disconcerting about their very existence. Indeed, most noneditorial articles on the population focus on the fact that returnees are frequently the victims of bullying, shut out of normal social relations, and deeply unhappy.

3.「日本人は、〜 な〜 原始時代の原始〜 ま、お猿に近い時の人間〜 ま、それか、日本の人の生活は、〜 木の実とか〜 根を食うたり〜 した。先祖がね。体質を持っているから、〜 ま、欧米なんかは、肉食の体質をずっと先祖から受け継いで、いるでしょう？」

4.「糖尿病になりやすいというか、たぶん、食べ物が日本人は日本の物を食べて、魚とかみそ汁とか、野菜を食べたりとかしてたのに、それで日本人の体のつくりに合った食べ物だったのに、違う文化がメインにになったので、合わないでしょ、体と食べ物がそれで糖尿になってると。」

5.「そうですね。なりやすいというか、やっぱり、何千年も何万年も日本人がしてきた食生活、体のつくりがそういうふうになってるので、過剰にたくさんお砂糖とか油とか、そういうものを摂るとなりやすい体なんだな、というところが思いますね。どうなのかな。実際はそういう話を聞いたような気がするんですけど。」

6.「だから私達は日本人だから、元々の日本人の食生活に少しまた、変えた方が良いのかなあ。ただ、もちろん、日本食がベストではないけども、日本人にとっては日本食が、もうちょっと、」

7.「それはやはり洋食でしょう。欧米化の食事でしょう。日本人本来の和食。」

8. See http://www.eiyoukeisan.com/calorie/gramphoto/zgaisyoku/bentou.html for a calorie breakdown of every bento option available from the four major national chains. (Japanese language.) Accessed May 2018.

9. See http://www.mcdonalds.co.jp/quality/basic_information/menu_info.php ?mid=1010 for basic hamburger on the market in Japan. (Japanese language.) Accessed May 2018.

10. See http://www.mcdonalds.co.jp/quality/basic_information/menu_info.php ?mid=1700 for nutritional information. (Japanese language.) Accessed October 2010.

11. The smallest *donburi* at the popular chain Yoshinoya contains 667 calories. The more common middle size contains 837 calories, and the special set contains 1,008 calories. See http://www.yoshinoya.com/menu/don/gyudon.html. (Japanese language.) Accessed May 2018.

12. See http://www.aji1000.co.jp/#menu. (Japanese language.) Accessed May 2018.

13. See http://www.eiyoukeisan.com/calorie/gramphoto/zryouri/ramen.html. (Japanese language.) Accessed May 2018.

14.「まあ一言で言えば欧米化になるんじゃないのかな。うん。うん。だから今言ってるのはその、スローフード、であの一日本食に戻したい . . .」

15.「前は、どういうのかな、肉食じゃなくって、あの、米とか野菜とかの食事だったからカロリーが低くて。で、それで、あの、肝臓の方が、肝臓っていうのかインシュリンを作るすい臓か。そっちの方の機能が小っちゃくても大丈夫だったんだけど、今の食生活って肉とか高カロリーの食事ばっかりで。で、アメリカとか欧米の人っていうのはそれをずーっとしてきて遺伝的に堪えられる体になってるんだと思うんだけど。」

16.「なりやすい。日本人は昔はそんなスイートとか肉はあんまり食べなかったので、インシュリンが必要でなかった。More than thousands 日本人は took rice 米を食べてましたから。インシュリン分泌が必要でなかった。それが第二 after the World War the Second, we began to eat meat and sweets. They need more insulin but they don't secrete insulin to meet that. 非常にアメリカ人、ヨーロッパ人に比べて糖尿病になり易い、日本人は。」

17.「節約遺伝子、倹約遺伝子という、元々島国だったから、食べなくていいような、私もそうなっていますけど、食べなくてもいいような人たちが生き残っている。」

「患者さんにその遺伝の事を説明しますか?」

「します。あの、痛風、高尿酸血でも説明します。高脂血症でも説明します。だから患者さんの中にはまあ、いろんなタイプがありますけど、自分が悪いんだと思っている方も結構おられるんですよ。そうでなくて、遺伝的な物もあるんですよー」

18.「最近日本で糖尿病が増えているんですけど、どうしてだと思いますか? 」

「何だろう。食習慣も関係してるんかな、と思うんですよね。あの、ま、その。食習慣じゃないんですか。結構あの、何? 食べ、肥満。食べ過ぎたり。うん、すごく沢山食べたりしてるから。それから日本食、日本食キチッと食べればねすごい、日本の食事はいいと思うんだけど、外国のハンバーガーとかね。」

19.「和食のようなバランスだったらいいんだけど、どうしても油使って、料理することが有るから。」

20.「ご飯と、後、魚と、というのは、やっぱり基本で良いと思うんですね。やっぱり油を減らすということだと思う。」

21.「もうここ最近はその健康、健康で日本食がやっぱりいいよって言って見直されてはきてるけれども。こう、流れ的には和食の文化からその欧米化っていうか、ねえ、洋食の文化の方がもう多くなってきてる。もう若い世代なんか特に、あの、和食のおかずよりも洋食、パン、ま子供達でいえばハンバーグだとかエビフライだとか。そういう系の方が好きで。だから好きだから親もそっちを作るし。で、そういう子達が大っきくなると和食のいいところは、こう、もう、何て言うのかな、覚えられずに自分の好きな物だけを食べていってたら結局そうなるのかなっていう気はするんですけど。うん。なんか、まあ、日本人はお魚をよく食べる人種ですよね。だけど若い子達は今の日本人の若い子達はやっぱりお魚よりお肉が好きだし。」

22.「それは欧米化の食生活と運動不足と、それからストレスでしょうね。あの、オリエンタルメディシンの漢方薬とか針とか。ええと、その漢方のええと。。分かりやすいかな、疲れやすいっていうの、ききょうという、気が足りない、気がきょしている、気が足りない。要するに元気の気が足りないんで、電池で言えば充電の電池が切れてるような状態、切れかかっている状態の方が多いですね。疲れちゃって。で、なおかつイライラしたりとか、ストレスがあって、それがうまく巡らない。気ってのは全身を巡るんですけど、気がうまく巡らなくなっている人とかがすごく増えているんで、そうすると糖尿病になりやすい。だから、すごく人が多いと。まあ疲れちゃう。それから、イライラストレスを抱えている方が多いんで、糖尿病がすごく増えてるなあっていう印象はありますけど。」

Chapter Five

1. Not speaking about oneself personally is a point of etiquette, not a security measure.

2.「目が会った方とは会釈する。」

3.「挨拶を欠かさない。」

4.「患者様のお顔とお名前は出来るだけ早く覚える。」

5. This refers to a formal verb form used in polite speech. 「言葉使いは "です" "ます" 調で話す。」

6.「どんなに忙しくとも、柔らかい、女性らしい応対に心がける。」

7.「患者様の苦情にはまず、"申し訳ございません" とお詫びしてから、具体的にお答えする。直接に反論は絶対にしないこと。」

8.「患者と医師の関係は、施されるものと施すもの、弱者と強者といった雰囲気にならないようお願いいたします。患者さんへの態度、言葉遣いには特に注意し

てください。医療はサービス業としてみられつつある世の流れを認識して、診療にあたるようお願いします。当院の「患者さんの権利擁護宣言」をご参照下さい。」

9.「結構日本では、やっぱり医師からこうしなさい、ああしなさいと言われる方が好きな人がまだ、結構お年が入った方の中では多いなってすごく思います。それから、かなり若い 20 代位とか、あと結構いろいろこうインテリジェンスが高い方とかは、最近インターネットとかで調べて自分はこういう風な治療がしたいとか、こういう薬が出ている筈ですけどどうですか、というのがたまにいらっしゃるんですでど、その他の方は、逆にこっちがこれとこれがあるんですけどどうしましょうか、って言った場合に自分じゃ全くわからないから全部決めて欲しい、って言われた方が多いですね。」

10.「要するに運動量から計算した。メッツ (METS) を計算して、運動処方というね、を出しますけどね。で処方は何ですかね? exercise を prescription を出しまして。うん。だからそれは具体的に計算して、これぐらいするとこれぐらいカロリーが減るっていうのは、患者には出しますけど自分は非常に大まかです。」

11.「まあみんなよく知っていますけどね。知識は結構特にインターネットとかで、病気の知識をすごい知ってる人と知らない人とまあ差がありますけどもね。世界的な傾向かと思うんですけど、医者が知ってるべきことでも、普通の一般の人でもインターネットで調べれば、検索すれば、何でも分かるんです。」

12.「私的には書物で勉強する方が多いんですが、一般の人たちはもう何でもこの頃インターネットで。もうインターネットという携帯で、何でもできる時代で、特に若い人なんかは。」

13.「ええ。あの〜　まあ食事療法が、まあ、運動療法より食事療法の起用が高い。まあ、85% が食事療法によるということと、後はやっぱり、あの〜　、なかなかですね、あのこうしようと言ってもなかなか守ってくれないので、あの〜　、私良くやってるのは、体重を 1 日 4 回体重を計って貰ってですね、グラフにして貰って、それを見て、もう後は患者さんが、どう感じるかと、自分で健康を、あの〜管理して貰うという、いわゆるセルフコントロールっていう、まあ、そういうプログラムじゃないと難しいと思ってますので、私からは体重を付けて下さいとしか言わないんですけどね。それを見て、どう判断して、どういう風に改善するかは、まあ、患者に任せます。」

14.「お薬だけ、あの、お薬を飲まれる方のみであればやはり、そのお薬に頼るのではなくって、えー、食事がまず基本だと。いう事を一番によく言っておかないと、結構飲み薬を飲むと「あ、これで私は大丈夫」という安心感がでちゃうんですよね。」

15.「治療を一番継続しなきゃいけないっていうのが難しいケースがやっぱりありますね。入院された方は短期間がんばれば直ると思っている方もいるので、そうじゃなくて、まあ病気は病気なんだけど、これはあなたの体質なのでたとえ運動や食事療法良くして、血糖が下がりやすくなっても、同じようにお菓子を食べれば血糖は上がるし、病気が治るわけではないんですよっていうのが、なかなか糖尿病は治らないんですよっていうのが、なかなか説明してもちょっと伝わってないのかなと思いますね。」

Chapter Six

1. 「病気にならないために、一番いい生活習慣な何だと思いますか？」
「規則正しい生活ですか。はい。」
「具体的にどういう意味ですか？」
「毎朝決まった時間に起きる、決まった時間にご飯を食べる、栄養のバランスのいい食事を摂る、規則正しい生活リズム。」

2. "That" refers to westernization—the adoption of Western food and habits and the rejection of traditional Japanese food.

3. 「それと不規則。不規則なのがいけないんじゃない。不規則わかります？ 要するに、あの、あの、朝・昼・夕をキチッと食べなくて朝・晩にしたりとか、間で食べたりとか、あのどういうか、決まって食べないか。それかすごく遅く、夜遅くに食事をするとか。そういう食事の乱れも関係してるんかな、とは思うんですけどね。うーん。」

4. I had recently participated in a Shinto religious pilgrimage with the family to ensure the prosperity of their agricultural endeavors. The trip required the five of us to spend hours driving overnight to a mountain of religious significance, then don pilgrims' robes and begin climbing the mountain in the rain at 2 A.M. so as to reach the shrine that marked the gateway to the holy part of the mountain by 5 A.M. We then took sips of ceremonial sake and climbed another three hours in the rain to reach the shrine at the peak, be blessed, and eat some rice, pickles, and miso soup before descending. I was teased for being an enthusiastic climber but slow at descending because I had not conserved energy, so that Akiko and Daisuke, both in their sixties, nearly beat me. "She goes up like an energetic kid, but goes down like a grandmother!" they repeated to every curious pilgrim we passed on the way down, and then to half the town after we returned home.

5. 「規則ただしい生活、睡眠、休養、栄養。」
「広告みたいですね。」
「言っても守りません。」
「あと睡眠十分とって、栄養摂って。」
「言う事と実行はイコールじゃないね。まあみんなそうだと思いますけど。」

6. 「あんまり口では言わなかったと思いますけど、だいたい同じ時間に起こして、朝はきちんとタンパク質とか、ビタミンとかでんぷん質とか。で、学校行っても頭が働かないから、ちゃんと炭水化物も食べなきゃだめよ、って言って、とりあえず朝はきちんと食べさせていくようには心がけてはいました。それで夜は、もう晩ご飯終わったらあとは何も食べない。。。早く寝るようには言って、ちゃんとだいたいそういうことだけに気をつけたかな。あとはあんまり、あの、こっちもルーズですから。もうルーズに育ててきました。」

7. 「私は不規則だったの。散髪屋。ちょっと 5 分お待ちください、ってお客さん来れたらはいってね。もうご飯に味噌汁かけてササササーっていって、ほいで直ぐ行って仕事でしょ。5 分言ったらね 7 分でも待たすの嫌な方だから。。。だからなあいい加減ズルズルでこうやって、うーん、寝とけばいいみたいな事は出来ないしね。忙しかったから。今は暇にはなってるけどね。」

8.「ただ規則正しい生活が多分いいと思いますね。で、あまりいっぱいおいしいものを食べないほうがいいかな。」

9.「でも、糖尿病の考えは全然なかった。」

10.「だから、初めて糖尿病と聞いた時、もう既に余り良くないって、その糖尿病のスタートがなかった私。ちょっと大分悪かったでしょ？だから、え〜 っ！！と思って、だから目が見えなくなっちゃ嫌だとか、旅行に歩いて行けなくなったら嫌だとか、それは凄く思った。」

11.「もちろん、1番は私のDNA？と思う。　DNAプラス何？私の食べることとストレスと。もちろん、ず〜　っと前から、私のライフスタイルが良くないのは自分で1番良く知っていたから。」

12.「うん、私はまだ、はっきり糖尿病と言えないけど、でも、気をつけないと、糖尿病になってしまうから。だから、食べ物や、運動に気をつけましょうと。と言われて。で、私は糖尿病になりたくなかったので、一生懸命努力しました。で、今のところは。なので、完全に糖尿病ではない。私の年齢からすると、6.0　くらいまで抑えてたら良いでしょうと、言われました。年齢、若かったけども、私ももう、六十六に成りますから、シクスティーシックス。ま、これぐらいで。」

13.「糖尿病って言われるのが、私嫌で。だから呼びになると、食べ物に、すごい制限が有りますよね。これだけって、それがつらいから、糖尿病と言われたくないので、自分で抑えて、してます。」

14.「仕事上、かかっている人をよくみるから。」

15.「死にいたる病気なので。」

16.「糖尿病にならないように、どうすればいいと思いますか？」

17.「自己管理・（検診）してる」

18.「甘いものを食べ過ぎないようにしています。」

19.「毎月1回血液検査。血糖値に異常はないと思う。」

20.「ああ、そうですね。私は、あの〜 、ファミリーヒストリーと言いますかね。あの、多いので、おそらくなると思います。（笑い声）」

21.「やっぱり日常生活で意識をしなかったら、食生活で脂の摂取量とか、かなり多くなってしまうし、糖の摂取量というのもやっぱり多い。普通あのポカリスウェットとかああいう飲み物、スポーツドリンクもペットボトルにもうこれぐらい砂糖が入っているというのが、私も医者になるまで知らなかったので、みんなもほとんど知らないですよね。だから私はまあ知識があるのでなるべくそういうおやつなんかは、昔は好きでしたけど食べないようにして、油物もなるべく控えるようにして、運動はもともとあまり好きじゃないのでできないんですけど、まあ職場でなるべく階段を使うようにとか、ずっとそれを継続してやるのも難しいんですけど、時々思い立ってまた気をつけようっていう感じで。気をつけようと自分はしてますね。」

22.「自分の家族のために、糖尿病について、心配しますか？」

　　「家は、別に、ま、あの、規則正しい食事と、バランスの良い食事とかは、心掛けていますが、特別 . . . 　ま、糖尿病ってことに限っては、全体的な健康、を考えています。ですけど、そんなに完璧では無いので、心掛けてはいますけど、完璧では無いです。気持ちは。」

Methodological Appendix

1. Not Hosekijima.

2. The suburban private hospital at which I was based gave me the title "visiting international researcher" (*gaikokujin kengakuin*). My identification at the urban welfare hospital, on the other hand, read "intern" (*kenshuuin*). In other contexts I was typically introduced as a visiting international researcher from the sociology department at Okayama University (*Okadai no shakaigakubu no gaikokujin kenkyuuin*).

Works Cited

Abraham, John. 2009. "Partial Progress: Governing the Pharmaceutical Industry and the NHS, 1948–2008." *Journal of Health Politics, Policy and Law* 34 (6): 931–77.

———. 2010. "Pharmaceuticalization of Society in Context: Theoretical, Empirical and Health Dimensions." *Sociology* 44 (4): 603–22.

Abrums, Mary. 2000. "'Jesus Will Fix It after Awhile': Meanings and Health." *Social Science and Medicine* 50: 89–105.

AbuSabha, Rayane, and Cheryl Achterberg. 1997. "Review of Self-Efficacy and Locus of Control for Nutrition- and Health-Related Behavior." *Journal of the American Dietetic Association* 97 (10): 1122–32.

Allan, Janet D. 1998. "Explanatory Models of Overweight among African American, Euro-American, and Mexican American Women." *Western Journal of Nursing Research* 20 (1): 45–66.

Amemiya, S., and T. Hoshino. 2013. "The Worldwide Standardization of Hemoglobin A1c Measurement: The Current Statement from the Japan Diabetes Society and the Issues To Be Solved." [In Japanese.] *Rinsho Byori* 61 (7): 594–601.

American Diabetes Association. 2002. *The Impact of Diabetes.*

———. 2003. *Direct and Indirect Costs of Diabetes in the United States.*

———. 2007. "2007 National Diabetes Fact Sheet." Available online: http://www .diabetes.org/diabetes-basics/diabetes-statistics/. Accessed December 2010.

American Medical Association. 2009. *Physician Characteristics and Distribution in the U.S., 2009.* Chicago: American Medical Association.

Andersen, Ronald M. 1995. "Revisiting the Behavioral Model and Access to Medical Care: Does It Matter?" *Journal of Health and Social Behavior* 36: 1–10.

Anderson, Ronald M., and Martha Mitchell Funnell. 2000. *The Art of Empowerment: Stories and Strategies for Diabetes Educators.* Alexandria, VA: American Diabetes Association.

Anderson, Ronald M., Martha M. Funnell, James T. Fitzgerald, and David G. Marrero. 2000. "The Diabetes Empowerment Scale: A Measure of Psychosocial Self-Efficacy." *Diabetes Care* 23 (6): 739–43.

Aneshensel, Carol S. 1992. "Social Stress: Theory and Research." *Annual Review of Sociology* 18: 15–38.

Angelucci, Patricia. 1995. "Cultural Diversity: Health Belief Systems." *Nursing Management* 26 (8): 72.

Armstrong-Hough, Mari. 2015. "Origins of Difference: Professionalization, Power, and Mental Hygiene in Canada and the United States." *American Review of Canadian Studies* 45 (2): 208–25.

———. "ADHD in Japan: A Sociological Perspective." In *Global Perspectives on ADHD: Social Dimensions of Diagnosis and Treatment in Sixteen Countries,* edited by

Meredith R. Bergey, Angela M. Filipe, Peter Conrad, and Ilina Singh, 261–69. Baltimore, MD: Johns Hopkins University Press.

Arnason, Johann P. 1997. *Social Theory and Japanese Experience*. London: Kegan Paul International.

Balshem, Martha. 1993. *Cancer in the Community: Class and Medical Authority*. Washington, DC: Smithsonian Institution Press.

Bay, Alexander R. 2012. *Beriberi in Modern Japan: The Making of a National Disease*. Rochester, NY: University of Rochester Press.

Bandura, Albert. 1977. "Self-Efficacy: Toward a Unifying Theory of Behavioral Change." *Psychological Review* 84 (2): 191–215.

Barber, Benjamin. 1996. *Jihad vs. McWorld: How Globalism and Tribalism Are Reshaping the World*. New York: Ballantine Books.

Barton, Josh, Kevin Dew, Anthony Dowell, Nicolette Sheridan, Timothy Kenealy, Lindsay Macdonald, Barbara Docherty, Rachel Tester, Debbie Raphael, Lesley Gray, and Maria Stubbe. 2016. "Patient Resistance as a Resource: Candidate Obstacles in Diabetes Consultations." *Sociology of Health and Illness* 38 (7): 1151–66.

Beaser, Richard S., and Amy P. Campbell. 2005. *The Joslin Guide to Diabetes*. New York: Simon & Schuster.

Becker, Gay, and Sharon Kaufman. 1995. "Managing and Uncertain Illness Trajectory in Old Age: Patients' and Physicians' Views of Stroke." *Medical Anthropology Quarterly* 9: 165–87.

Becker, Marshall H., Lois A. Maiman, John P. Kirscht, Don P. Haifner, and Robert H. Drachman. 1977. "The Health Belief Model and Prediction of Dietary Compliance: A Field Experiment." *Journal of Health and Social Behavior* 18: 348–66.

Bell, Susan E., and Anne E. Figert. 2012. "Medicalization and Pharmaceuticalization at the Intersections: Looking Backward, Sideways and Forward." *Social Science and Medicine* 75: 775–83.

Ben-Ari, Eyal, Brian Moeran, and James Valentine, eds. 1992. *Unwrapping Japan: Society and Culture in Anthropological Perspective*. Honolulu: University of Hawaii Press.

Bergen, Clara, and Tanya Stivers. 2013. "Patient Disclosure of Medical Misdeeds." *Journal of Health and Social Behavior* 54 (2): 221–40.

Beukers, H., A. M. Luyendijk-Elshout, M. E. van Opstall, and F. Vos. 1991. "Red-Hair Medicine: Dutch-Japanese Medical Relations." *Nieuwe Nederlandse bijdragen tot de geschiedenis der geneeskunde en der natuurwetenschappen* 36: 1–114.

Biehl, João. 2004. "Life of the Mind: The Interface of Psychopharmaceuticals, Domestic Economies, and Social Abandonment." *American Ethnologist* 31 (4): 475–96.

Boaz, Noel T. 2002. *Evolving Health: The Origins of Illness and How the Modern World Is Making Us Sick*. New York: John Wiley & Sons.

Boli, John, and George M. Thomas. 1997. "World Culture in the World Polity: A Century of International Non-governmental Organization." *American Sociological Review* 62: 171–90.

Borovoy, Amy, and Janet Hine. 2008. "Managing the Unmanageable: Elderly Russian Jewish Émigrés and the Biomedical Culture of Diabetes Care." *Medical Anthropology Quarterly* 22 (1): 1–26.

Bowers, J. Z. 1979. "The Adoption of German Medicine in Japan: the Decision and the Beginning." *Bulletin of the History of Medicine* 53 (1): 57–80.

Broom, Dorothy, and Andrea Whittaker. 2004. "Controlling Diabetes, Controlling Diabetics: Moral Language in the Management of Diabetes Type 2." *Social Science and Medicine* 58: 2371–82.

Brown, P. 1995. "Naming and Framing: The Social Construction of Diagnosis and Illness." *Journal of Health and Social Behavior* 35: 34–52.

Bureau of Labor Statistics. 2010. *Occupational Outlook Handbook, 2010–2011 Edition.*

Burns, Susan. 2003. *Before the Nation: Kokugaku and the Imagining of Community in Early Modern Japan.* Durham, NC: Duke University Press.

Bush, James P. 1988. "Job Satisfaction, Powerlessness, and Locus of Control." *Western Journal of Nursing Research* 10 (6): 718–31.

Centers for Disease Control and Prevention. 2011. "National Diabetes Factsheet 2011."

Cerimagic, Zlata. 2004. "Self-Reported Medication Adherence among Patients with Diabetes." Ph.D. dissertation, University of Rhode Island.

Chan, Juliana C. N., Vasanti Malik, Weiping Jia, Takashi Kadowaki, Chittaranjan S. Yajnik, Kun-Ho Yoon, and Frank B. Hu. 2009. "Diabetes in Asia: Epidemiology, Risk Factors, and Pathophysiology." *Journal of the American Medical Association* 301 (20): 2129–40.

Chapell, K. 2002. "Diabetes: A New Look at a Killer Disease." *Ebony* 57 (5): 121–24.

Charmaz, Kathy. 1983. "The Grounded Theory Method: An Explication and Interpretation." In *Contemporary Field Research*, edited by Robert M. Emerson, 109–26. Boston: Little, Brown.

———. 1990. "'Discovering' Chronic Illness: Using Grounded Theory." *Social Science Medicine* 20: 1161–72.

———. 1991. *Good Days, Bad Days: The Self in Chronic Illness and Time.* New Brunswick, NJ: Rutgers University Press.

———. 2000. "Grounded Theory: Objectivist and Constructivist Methods." In *Handbook of Qualitative Research*, edited by Norman K. Denzin and Yvonna S. Lincoln, 509–35. Thousand Oaks, CA: Sage.

Chesla, Catherine. A., Kevin M. Chun, and Christine M. L. Kwan. 2009. "Cultural and Family Challenges to Managing Type 2 Diabetes in Immigrant Chinese Americans." *Diabetes Care* 32 (10): 1812–16.

Chesla, Catherine A., Marilyn M. Skaff, Robert J. Bartz, Joseph T. Mullan, and Lawrence Fisher. 2000. "Differences in Personal Models among Latinos and European Americans." *Diabetes Care* 23 (12): 1780–85.

Clark, Noreen, and Molly Gong. 2000. "Management of Chronic Disease by Practitioners and Patients: Are We Teaching the Wrong Things?" *British Medical Journal* 320 (7234): 572–5.

Clarke, Adele E. 2010. "From the Rise of Medicine to Biomedicalization: U.S. Healthscapes and Iconography, Circa 1890–Present." In *Biomedicalization:*

Technoscience, Health, and Illness in the U.S., edited by Adele E. Clarke, Laura Mamo, Jennifer Ruth Fosket, Jennifer R. Fishman, and Janet K. Shim, 104–46. Durham, NC: Duke University Press.

Clarke, Adele E., Laura Mamo, Jennifer Ruth Fosket, Jennifer R. Fishman, and Janet K. Shim, eds. 2010. *Biomedicalization: Technoscience, Health, and Illness in the U.S.* Durham, NC: Duke University Press.

Clarke, Adele E., Janet K. Shim, Laura Mamo, Jennifer Ruth Fosket, and Jennifer R. Fishman. 2003. "Biomedicalization: Technoscientific Transformations of Health, Illness, and U.S. Biomedicine." *American Sociological Review* 68 (2): 161–94.

CNN. 2009. "Best Jobs in America." Online. https://money.cnn.com/magazines /moneymag/bestjobs/2009/snapshots/4.html Accessed 1/24/2011.

Cohen, Marlene Z., Toni Tripp-Reimer, Christopher Smith, Bernard Sorofman, and Sonja Lively. 1994. "Explanatory Models of Diabetes: Patient Practitioner Variation." *Social Science and Medicine* 38: 59–66.

Cohen-Cole, Steven A. 1991. *The Medical Interview: The Three Function Approach.* St. Louis: Year Book Medical Pub.

Conrad, Peter. 1985. "The Meaning of Medications: Another Look at Compliance." *Social Science and Medicine* 20 (1): 29–37.

———. 2005. "The Shifting Engines of Medicalization." *Journal of Health and Social Behavior* 46 (1): 3–14.

Conrad, P., and V. Leiter. 2004. "Medicalization, Markets and Consumers." *Journal of Health and Social Behavior* 45: 158–76.

Conrad, Peter, and Joseph W. Schneider. 1992. *Deviance and Medicalization: From Badness to Sickness.* Philadelphia: Temple University Press.

Critchley, Julia A., Blanca I. Restrepo, Katharina Ronacher, Anil Kapur, Andrew A. Bremer, Larry S. Schlesinger, Randall Basaraba, Hardy Kornfeld, and Reinout van Crevel. 2017. "Defining a Research Agenda to Address the Converging Epidemics of Tuberculosis and Diabetes. Part 1: Epidemiology and Clinical Management." *Chest* 152 (1):165–73.

Crossette, Barbara. 2001. "U.N. Board Says Legal Drug Use Increases in Rich Countries." *New York Times*, February 21, 2001, A.9.

Dale, Peter. 2012. *The Myth of Japanese Uniqueness.* London: Routledge.

———. 1988. "The Myth of Japanese Uniqueness Revisited." Nissan Institute of Japanese Studies.

Davidson, Mayer B., and Debra L. Gordon. 2009. *The Complete Idiot's Guide to Diabetes.* Indianapolis, IN: Alpha Books.

Davies, P. 2007. "The Predictability of Research in Chronic Illness." *Journal of Epidemiology and Community Health* 61 (6): 467.

Dickinson, S., S. Colagiuri, E. Faramus, P. Petocz, and J. C. Brand-Miller. 2002. "Postprandial Hyperglycemia and Insulin Sensitivity Differ Among Lean Young Adults of Different Ethnicities." *The Journal of Nutrition* 132 (9): 2574–79.

Doi, Takeo. 1981. *The Anatomy of Dependence: The Key Analysis of Japanese Behavior.* Translated by John Bester. 2nd ed. Tokyo: Kodansha International.

Douglas, Mary. 1966. *Purity and Danger.* Reprint edition 2002. London: Routledge Classics.

Duignan, R. (2012). Saving 10,000: Winning a War on Suicide in Japan. A Duignan & Astier Documentary Film. Boomachine Studios, Tokyo, Japan. Retrieved from http://www.saving10000.com/.

Dunkley, Alison J., Danielle H. Bodicoat, Colin J. Greaves, Claire Russell, Thomas Yates, Melanie J. Davies, and Kamlesh Khunti. 2014. "Diabetes Prevention in the Real World: Effectiveness of Pragmatic Lifestyle Interventions for the Prevention of Type 2 Diabetes and of the Impact of Adherence to Guideline Recommendations: A Systematic Review and Meta-Analysis." *Diabetes Care* 37 (4): 922–33.

Egede, Leonard E. 2004. "Diabetes, Major Depression, and Functional Disability among U.S. Adults." *Diabetes Care* 27 (2): 421–8.

Ellis, Jonathan, Ian Mulligan, James, Rowe, and David L. Sackett. 1995. "Inpatient General Medicine Is Evidence Based." *Lancet* 346 (8972): 407–10.

Fadiman, Anne. 1997. *The Spirit Catches You and You Fall Down: A Hmong Child, Her American Doctors, and the Collision of Two Cultures.* New York: Farrar, Straus and Giroux.

Felder, Kay, Ulrike Felt, and Michael Penkler. 2015. "Caring for Evidence: Research and Care in an Obesity Outpatient Clinic." *Medical Anthropology* 35 (5): 404–18.

Ferzacca, Steve. 2000. "'Actually, I Don't Feel that Bad': Managing Diabetes and the Clinical Encounter." *Medical Anthropology Quarterly* 14 (1): 28–50.

Finkler, Kaja. 2004. "Biomedicine Globalized and Localized: Western Medical Practices in an Outpatient Clinic of a Mexican Hospital." *Social Science and Medicine* 59 (10): 2037.

Ford, Daniel E. 2008. "Optimizing Outcomes for Patients with Depression and Chronic Medical Illnesses." *American Journal of Medicine* 121 (11B): S38–S44.

Foucault, Michel. 1963. *The Birth of the Clinic: An Archaeology of Medical Perception.* Reprint edition 1994. London: Vintage.

———. 1965. *Madness and Civilization.* London: Tavistock.

Fox, J. B., and C. L. Richards. 2010. "Vital Signs: Health Insurance Coverage and Health Care Utilization—United States, 2006–2009 and January–March 2010." *Morbidity and Mortality Weekly Report* 59 (44): 1448–54.

Frank, Robert, and Gunnar Stollberg. 2004. "Conceptualizing Hybridization: On the Diffusion of Asian Medical Knowledge to Germany." *International Sociology* 19 (1): 71–88.

Frühstück, Sabine. 2005. "Male Anxieties: Nerve Force, Nation, and the Power of Sexual Knowledge." *Journal of the Royal Asiatic Society* 15 (1):71–88.

Fuyuno, Ichiko. 2011. "Japan: Will the Sun Set on Kampo?" *Nature* 480 (7378): S96–S96.

Gage-Bouchard, Elizabeth A. 2017. "Culture, Styles of Institutional Interactions, and Inequalities in Healthcare Experiences." *Journal of Health and Social Behavior* 58 (2): 147–65.

George, Linda K. 1996. "Social Factors and Illness." In *Handbook of Aging and the Social Sciences,* 4th ed., edited by Robert H. Binstock and Linda K. George, 229–52. San Diego, CA: Academic Press.

Gill, Virginia T., Anita Pomerantz, and Paul Denvir. 2010. "Pre-Emptive Resistance: Patients' Participation in Diagnostic Sense-Making Activities." *Sociology of Health and Illness* 32 (1): 1–20.

Gill, P., A. C. Dowell, R. D. Neal, N. Smith, P. Heywood, and A. E. Wilson. 1996. "Evidence Based General Practice: a Retrospective Study of Interventions in One Training Practice." *British Medical Journal* 312: 819–21.

Glaser, Barney G. 1992. *Basics of Grounded Theory Analysis.* Mill Valley, CA: Sociology Press.

Glaser, Barney, and Anselm Strauss. 1967. *The Discovery of Grounded Theory.* Chicago: Aldine.

Glasgow, Russell E. and Robert M. Anderson. 1999. "In Diabetes Care, Moving from Compliance to Adherence Is Not Enough. Something Entirely Different Is Needed." *Diabetes Care* 22 (12): 2090–2.

Glasgow, Russell E., Sarah E. Hampson, Lisa A. Strycker, and Laurie Ruggiero. 1997. "Personal-Model Beliefs and Social Environmental Barriers Related to Diabetes Self-Management." *Diabetes Care* 20: 556–61.

Gluckman, Peter, and Mark Hanson. 2006. *Mismatch: The Lifestyle Diseases Timebomb.* Oxford: Oxford University Press.

Glumer, Charlotte, Dorte Vistisen, Knut Borch-Johnsen, and Stephen Colagiuri. 2006. "Risk Scores for Type 2 Diabetes Can Be Applied in Some Populations but Not All." *Diabetes Care* 29 (2): 410–14.

Gonzalez, Jeffrey S., Lawrence Fisher, and William H. Polonsky. 2011. "Depression in Diabetes: Have We Been Missing Something Important?" *Diabetes Care* 34 (1): 236–9.

Goodman, Roger. 1992. "Deconstructing an Anthropological Text: A 'Moving' Account of Returnee Schoolchildren in Contemporary Japan." In *Unwrapping Japan: Society and Culture in Anthropological Perspective,* edited by Eyal Ben-Ari, Brian Moeran, and James Valentine, 121–38. Honolulu: University of Hawaii Press.

Greene, Jeremy A. 2007. *Prescribing By Numbers: Drugs and the Definition of Disease.* Baltimore, MD: Johns Hopkins University Press.

Gregg, E., K. Kirtland, B. Cadwell, N. Burrows, L. Barker, T. Thompson, L. Geiss, and L. Pan. 2010. "Estimated County-Level Prevalence of Diabetes and Obesity-United States, 2007." *Journal of the American Medical Association* 303 (10): 933–5.

Haberman, Clyde. 1988. "Japanese Are Special Types, They Explain." *New York Times.* March 6. http://www.nytimes.com/1988/03/06/weekinreview/the-world-japanese-are-special-types-they-explain.html. Accessed May 2018.

Halanych, Jewell H., Monika M. Safford, Wendy C. Keys, Sharina D. Person, James M. Shikany, Young-Il Kim, Robert M. Centor, and Jeroan J. Allison. 2007. "Burden of Comorbid Medical Conditions and Quality of Diabetes Care." *Diabetes Care* 30 (12): 2999–3004.

Hall, Peter, and David Soskice, eds. 2001. *Varieties of Capitalism: The Institutional Foundations of Comparative Advantage.* Oxford: Oxford University Press.

Hamilton, Gary G., and Nicole Woolsey Biggart. 1988. "Market, Culture, and Authority: A Comparative Analysis of Management and Organization in the Far East." *American Journal of Sociology* 94: S52–S94.

Hampson, Sarah E. 1997. "Illness Representations and the Self Management of Diabetes." In *Perceptions of Health and Illness: Current Research and Applications,* edited by Keith J. Petrie and John Weinman, 323–48. Amsterdam: Harwood Academic Publishers.

Hampson, Sarah E., Russell E. Glasgow, and Lyn S. Foster. 1995. "Personal Models of Diabetes Among Older Adults: Relationship to Self-Management and Other Variables." *Diabetes Education* 21: 300–7.

Hampson, Sarah E., Russell E. Glasgow, and Deborah J. Toobert. 1990. "Personal Models of Diabetes and Their Relations to Self-Care Activities." *Health Psychology* 9: 632–46.

Harris, Maureen I. 2000. "Health Care and Health Status and Outcomes for Patients with Type 2 Diabetes." *Diabetes Care* 23 (6): 754–8.

Harris, Rachel, and Margaret W. Linn. 1985. "Health Beliefs, Compliance, and Control of Diabetes Mellitus." *Southern Medical Journal* 78 (2): 162–6.

Hayashi, Seino. 2009. 「脳に悪い7つの習慣」 [*Seven Habits that Are Bad for Your Brain.*] Tokyo: Gentosha Publishing.

Hayashino, Yasuaki, Satoru Tsujii, and Hitoshi Ishii. 2018. "Association of Diabetes Therapy-Related Quality of Life and Physical Activity Levels in Patients with Type 2 Diabetes Receiving Medication Therapy: The Diabetes Distress and Care Registry at Tenri (DDCRT 17)." *Acta Diabetologica* 55 (2): 165–73.

Henry, Lester, and Kirk A. Johnson. 1993. *The Black Health Library Guide to Diabetes.* New York: Henry Holt.

Heritage, John and Douglas W. Maynard. 2006. "Problems and Prospects in the Study of Physician-Patient Interaction: 30 Years of Research." *Annual Review of Sociology* 32 (1): 351–74.

Homei, Aya. 2006. "Birth Attendants in Meiji Japan: the Rise of a Medical Birth Model and the New Division of Labour." *Social History of Medicine* 19 (3): 407–24.

Hoshino, Kazumasa, ed. 1997. *Japanese and Western Bioethics: Studies in Moral Diversity.* Boston: Kluwer Academic Publishers.

House, J. S., J. M. Lepkowski, A. M. Kinney, R. P. Mero, R. C. Kessler, and A. R. Herzog. 1994. "The Social Stratification of Aging and Health." *Journal of Health and Social Behavior* 35: 213–34.

Hunt, Linda M., Meta Kreiner, and Howard Brody. 2012. "The Changing Face of Chronic Illness Management in Primary Care: A Qualitative Study of Underlying Influences and Unintended Outcomes." *Annals of Family Medicine* 10 (5): 452–60.

Hunt, L. M., J. C. D. Longworth, and K. B. de Voogd. 2002. *"If I Needed It, They Would Have Sent Me": Cancer Screening, Knowledge and Adherence Among Older Hispanic Women.* Julian Samora Research Institute, Michigan State University.

Hunt, Linda M., Miguel A. Valenzuela, and Jacqueline A. Pugh. 1998. "Porque Me Tocó a Mi? Mexican American Diabetes Patients' Causal Stories and Their Relationship to Treatment Behaviors." *Social Science and Medicine* 46 (8): 959–69.

Hunt, Linda, and Nedal H. Arar. 2001. "An Analytical Framework for Contrasting Patient and Provider Views of the Process of Chronic Disease Management." *Medical Anthropology Quarterly* 15 (3): 347–67.

Hunt, Nancy R. 1999. *A Colonial Lexicon of Birth Ritual, Medicalization, and Mobility in the Congo.* Durham, NC: Duke University Press.

Huntington, Samuel P. 1996. *The Clash of Civilizations and the Remaking of World Order*. New York: Simon & Schuster.

Hurley, Dan. 2010. *Diabetes Rising: How a Rare Disease Became a Modern Pandemic, and What to Do About It*. New York: Kaplan.

Iizuka, Toshiaki. 2007. "Experts' Agency Problems: Evidence From the Prescription Drug Market in Japan." *The RAND Journal of Economics* 38 (3): 844–62.

Ikeda, Kaori, Shimpei Fujimoto, Beth Morling, Shiho Ayano-Takahara, Andrew E. Carroll, Shin-ichi Harashima, Yukiko Uchida, and Nobuya Inagaki. 2014. "Social Orientation and Diabetes-Related Distress in Japanese and American Patients with Type 2 Diabetes." *PLOS ONE* 9 (10): e109323.

Ikeda, Kaori, Shimpei Fujimoto, Beth Morling, Shiho Ayano-Takahara, Shin-ichi Harashima, Yukiko Uchida, and Nobuya Inagaki. 2018. "Cross-Cultural Comparison of Predictors for Self-Care Behaviors in Patients with Type 2 Diabetes." *Journal of Diabetes Investigation*. Preprint before publication. DOI: 10.1111/jdi.12822.

Ikegami, Naoki and John C. Campbell. 1995. "Medical Care in Japan." *New England Journal of Medicine* 333: 1295–1299.

Ishibashi, M. 2013. "Introduction of the NGSP value in clinical practice and later." [In Japanese.] *Rinsho Byori* 61 (7): 602–6.

Iwabuchi, Koichi. 2002. *Recentering Globalization: Popular Culture and Japanese Transnationalism*. Durham, NC: Duke University Press.

Jannetta, Ann. 2007. *The Vaccinators: Smallpox, Medical Knowledge, and the "Opening" of Japan*. Stanford, CA: Stanford University Press.

Jansen, Marius B. 2002. *The Making of Modern Japan*. Cambridge, MA: Belknap Press of Harvard University Press.

Jezewski, Mary Ann, and Jane Poss. 2002. "Mexican Americans' Explanatory Model of Type 2 Diabetes." *Western Journal of Nursing Research* 24 (8): 840–58.

Judd, Deborah, Kathleen Sitzman, and G. Megan Davis. 2009. *A History of American Nursing: Trends and Eras*. New York: Jones & Bartlett.

Kashiwagi, Atsunori, et al. 2012. "International Clinical Harmonization of Glycated Hemoglobin in Japan: From Japan Diabetes Society to National Glycohemoglobin Standardization Program Values." *Journal of Diabetes Investigation* 3 (1): 39–40.

Kawaguchi, Teruko. 2007. "Certified Diabetes Expert Nurse and Nurse Educators in Japan." *Diabetes Research and Clinical Practice* 77 (3): S205–S207.

Kazufumi, Manabe, and Harumi Befu. 1993. "Japanese Cultural Identity: An Empirical Investigation of Nihonjinron." *Japanstudien* 4: 89–102.

Kelleher, David, and Sheila Hillier. 1996. *Researching Cultural Differences in Health*. London: Routledge.

Kennedy, Anne P., and Anne E. Rogers. 2002. "Improving Patient Involvement in Chronic Disease Management: The Views of Patients, GPs, and Specialists on a Guidebook for Ulcerative Colitis." *Patient Education and Counseling* 47 (3): 257–63.

Kerr, Alex. 2001. *Dogs and Demons: The Fall of Modern Japan*. London: Penguin.

Kimura, Masayo, Yoshinobu Kondo, Kazutaka Aoki, Jun Shirakawa, Hiroshi Kamiyama, Kazunari Kamiko, Shigeru Nakajima, and Yasuo Terauchi. 2018. "A Randomized Controlled Trial of a Mini Low-Carbohydrate Diet and an Energy-

Controlled Diet among Japanese Patients with Type 2 Diabetes." *Journal of Clinical Medicine Research* 10 (3): 182–8.

King, Elaine Boswell, David G. Schlundt, James W. Pichert, Charles K. Kinzer, and Barbara A. Backer. 2002. "Improving the Skills of Health Professionals in Engaging Patients in Diabetes-Related Problem Solving."*Journal of Continuing Education in the Health Professions* 22 (2): 94–102.

Kirk, Alison, Nanette Mutrie, Paul MacIntyre, and Miles Fisher. 2003. "Increasing Physical Activity in People with Type 2 Diabetes." *Diabetes Care* 26 (4): 1186–92.

Kleinman, Arthur. 1979. "Concepts and a Model for the Comparison of Medical Systems as Cultural Systems." *Social Science and Medicine* 23: 85–93.

———. 1981. *Patients and Healers in the Context of Culture.* Berkeley: University of California Press.

———. 1988. *The Illness Narratives: Suffering, Healing and the Human Condition.* New York: Basic Books.

———. 1995. *Writing at the Margin: Discourse between Anthropology and Medicine.* Berkeley: University of California Press.

Kosaka, Kinori, Mitsuihiko Noda, and Takeshi Kuzuya. 2005. "Prevention of Type 2 Diabetes by Lifestyle Intervention: A Japanese Trial in IGT Males." *Diabetes Research and Clinical Practice* 67 (2): 152–62.

Kreiner, Meta J. and Linda M. Hunt. 2014. "The Pursuit of Preventive Care for Chronic Illness: Turning Healthy People into Chronic Patients." *Sociology of Health & Illness* 36 (6): 870–84.

Lai, W. A., C.-Y. Lew-Ting, and W.-C. Chie. 2005. "How Diabetic Patients Think about and Manage Their Illness in Taiwan." *Diabetes Medicine* 22: 286–92.

Lamont, Michelle. 2000. *The Dignity of Working Men: Morality and the Boundaries of Race, Class, and Immigration.* Cambridge, MA: Harvard University Press.

Lange, Lori J., and John D. Piette. 2006. "Personal Models for Diabetes in Context and Patients' Health Status." *Journal of Behavioral Medicine* 29 (3): 239–53.

Leichter, Steven B. 2005. "Making Outpatient Care of Diabetes More Efficient: Analyzing Noncompliance." *Clinical Diabetes* 23 (4): 187–90.

Levinson, Wendy, and Nicole Lurie. 2004. "When Most Doctors Are Women: What Lies Ahead?" *Annals of Internal Medicine,* 141 (6): 471–4.

Light, Donald W. 2000a. "The Medical Profession and Organizational Change: From Professional Dominance to Countervailing Power." In *Handbook of Medical Sociology,* 5th ed., edited by Chloe E. Bird, Peter Conrad, and Allen M. Fremont, 201–16. Upper Saddle River, NJ: Prentice Hall.

———. 2000b. "The Sociological Character of Health Care Markets." In *Handbook of Social Studies in Health and Medicine,* edited by Gary L. Albrecht, Ray Fitzpatrick, and Susan C. Scrimshaw, . San Francisco: Sage.

Link, Bruce G., and Jo Phelan. 1995. "Social Conditions as Fundamental Causes of Disease." *Journal of Health and Social Behavior,* extra issue: 80–94.

Little, Randie R. and Curt L. Rohlfing. 2009. "HbA1c Standardization: Background, Progress and Current Issues." *Lab Medicine* 40 (6): 368–73.

Lock, Margaret. 1980. *East Asian Medicine in Urban Japan: Varieties of Medical Experience.* Berkeley: University of California Press.

———. 1995. *Encounters with Aging: Mythologies of Menopause in Japan and North America.* Berkeley: University of California Press.

Loewe, Ron, and Joshua Freeman. 2000. "Interpreting Diabetes Mellitus: Differences between Patient and Provider Models of Disease and Their Implications for Clinical Practice." *Culture, Medicine, and Psychiatry* 24: 379–401.

Lofland, John, and Lyn Lofland. 1984. *Analyzing Social Settings.* Belmont, CA: Wadsworth.

Long, Susan Orpett. 1987. "Health Care Providers: Technology, Policy, and Professional Dominance." In *Health, Illness, and Medical Care in Japan*, edited by Edward Norbeck and Margaret Lock, 66–88. Honolulu: University of Hawaii Press.

———. 2005. *Final Days: Japanese Culture and Choice at the End of Life.* Honolulu: University of Hawaii Press.

Lopez, Olivia. 2006. "Perceptions and Meanings of Type II Diabetes among Mexican American Farmworking Women." Ph.D. dissertation. University of Texas at Austin.

Low, Morris, ed. 2005. *Building a Modern Japan: Science, Technology, and Medicine in the Meiji Era and Beyond.* New York: Palgrave Macmillan.

Lutfey, Karen. 2005. "On Practices of 'Good Doctoring': Reconsidering the Relationship between Provider Roles and Patient Adherence." *Sociology of Health and Illness* 27 (4): 421–47.

Lutfey, Karen E., Stephen M. Campbell, Megan R. Renfrew, Lisa D. Marceau, Martin Roland, and John B. McKinlay. 2008. "How Are Patient Characteristics Relevant for Physicians' Clinical Decision Making in Diabetes? An Analysis of Qualitative Results from a Cross-National Factorial Experiment." *Social Science and Medicine* 67 (9): 1391–9.

Lutfey, Karen, and Jeremy Freese. 2005. "Toward Some Fundamentals of Fundamental Causality: Socioeconomic Status and Health in the Routine Clinic Visit for Diabetes." *American Journal of Sociology* 110 (5): 1326–72.

Lutfey, Karen, and W. J. Wishner. 1999. "Beyond 'Compliance' Is 'Adherence'. Improving the Prospect of Diabetes Care." *Diabetes Care* 22 (4): 635–9.

Ma, Defu, Hiromichi Sakai, Chihiro Wakabayashi, Jong-Sook Kwon, Yoonna Lee, Shuo Liu, Qiaoqin Wan, et al. 2017. "The Prevalence and Risk Factor Control Associated with Noncommunicable Diseases in China, Japan, and Korea." *Journal of Epidemiology / Japan Epidemiological Association* 27 (12): 568–73.

Maher, John. 1986. "The Development of English as an International Language of Medicine." *Applied Linguistics* 7 (2): 206–18.

Makhija, Mona V., Kwangsoo Kim, and Sandra D. Williamson. 1997. "Measuring Globalization of Industries Using a National Industry Approach: Empirical Evidence across Five Countries and over Time." *Journal of International Business Studies* 28 (4): 679–710.

Malek, Melanie Kay. 2006. "The Quest for Autonomy: Patient Decision-Making Behaviors in Type 2 Diabetes." Ph.D. dissertation. Texas State University—San Marcos.

Malnight, Thomas W. 1995. "Globalization of an Ethnocentric Firm: An Evolutionary Perspective." *Strategic Management Journal* 16 (2): 119–41.

Mann, Devin, Diego Ponieman, Howard Levanthal, and Ethan Halm. 2009. "Predictors of Adherence to Diabetes Medications: The Role of Disease and Medication Beliefs." *Journal of Behavioral Medicine* 32: 278–84.

Marcus, Erin. 2006. "When Young Doctors Strut Too Much of Their Stuff." *New York Times*, November 21, F5.

Maty, Sioban. C., Sherman A. James, and George A. Kaplan. 2010. "Life-Course Socioeconomic Position and Incidence of Diabetes Mellitus among Blacks and Whites: The Alameda County Study, 1965–1999." *American Journal of Public Health* 100 (1): 137.

Mayanagi, Makoto 真柳誠. 1998. 「医食同源の思想-成立と展開」 ["The Concept of *Ishokudogen*: Founding and Development."] *Sinica* 9 (10): 72–7.

McCarley, Patricia 2009. "Patient Empowerment and Motivational Interviewing: Engaging Patients to Self-Manage Their Own Care." *Nephrology Nursing Journal* 36 (4): 409.

McSweeney, Jean C., Janet D. Allan, and Kelly Mayo. 1997. "Exploring the Use of Explanatory Models in Nursing Research and Practice." *Journal of Nursing Scholarship* 29: 243–8.

McVeigh, Brian J. 2004. *Nationalisms of Japan: Managing and Mystifying Identity.* Lanham, MD: Rowman & Littlefield.

Mendenhall, Emily, Rebecca A. Seligman, Alicia Fernandez, and Elizabeth A. Jacobs. 2010. "Speaking Through Diabetes." *Medical Anthropology Quarterly* 24 (2): 220–39.

Mercado-Martinez, Francisco J., and Igor Martin Ramos-Herrera. 2002. "Diabetes: The Layperson's Theories of Causality." *Qualitative Health Research* 12 (6): 792–806.

Meyer, John W. 2000. "Globalization: Sources and Effects on National States and Societies." *International Sociology* 15: 233–48.

Mezuk, Briana, William W. Eaton, Sandra Albrecht, and Sherita Hill Golden. 2008. "Depression and Type 2 Diabetes over the Lifespan: A Meta-analysis." *Diabetes Care* 31 (12): 2383–90.

Miller, Delbert, and Neil Salkind. 2002. *Handbook of Research Design and Social Measurement.* 6th ed. Thousand Oaks, CA: Sage.

Min, Pyong Gap. 1992. "A Comparison of the Korean Minorities in China and Japan." *International Migration Review* 26 (1): 4–21.

MHLW (Ministry of Health, Labor and Welfare). 2007. 平成１７年国民健康・栄養調査報告. 厚生労働省.

———. 2010. 平成20年国民健康・栄養調査報告. 厚生労働省.

———. 2012. 平成22年国民健康・栄養調査報告. 厚生労働省.

———. 2014. 平成24年国民健康・栄養調査報告. 厚生労働省.

Ministry of Public Management, Home Affairs, Posts and Telecommunications. 2004. *White Paper: Information and Communications in Japan.* Tokyo: National Printing Bureau.

Ministry of Public Management, Home Affairs, Posts and Telecommunications. 2005. *White Paper: Information and Communications in Japan.* Tokyo: National Printing Bureau.

Mlinar, Zdravko. 1992. "Individuation and Globalization: The Transformation of Territorial Social Organization." In *Globalisation and Territorial Identities*, edited by Zdravko Mlinar, 1–14. Aldershot: Avebury.

Mölstad, Sigvard, Cecilia S. Lundborg, Anna-Karin Karlsson, and Otto Cars. 2002. "Antibiotic Prescription Rates Vary Markedly Between 13 European Countries." *Scandinavian Journal of Infectious Diseases* 34 (5): 366–71.

Morling, Beth, Shinobu Kitayama, and Yuri Miyamoto. 2003. "American and Japanese Women Use Different Coping Strategies during Normal Pregnancy." *Personality and Social Psychology Bulletin* 29 (12): 1533–46.

Morling, Beth, Yukiko Uchida, and Sandra Frentrup. 2015. "Social Support in Two Cultures: Everyday Transactions in the U.S. and Empathic Assurance in Japan." *PLOS ONE* 10 (6): e0127737.

Morris-Suzuki, Tessa. 1998. *Re-Inventing Japan: Time, Space, Nation*. Armonk, NY: M. E. Sharpe.

Nahm, Andrew C. 1988. *Korea: Tradition and Transformation—A History of the Korean People*. Elizabeth, NJ: Hollym International.

Nakagawa, Atsuo, Michael F. Grunebaum, Steven P. Ellis, Maria A. Oquendo, Haruo Kashima, Robert D. Gibbons, and J. John Mann. 2007. "Association of Suicide and Antidepressant Prescription Rates in Japan, 1999-2003." *Journal of Clinical Psychiatry* 68 (6): 908–16.

Nakamura, Raymond M. 1999. *Health in America: A Multicultural Perspective*. Boston: Allyn & Bacon.

Nakhnikian, George. 2004. "It Ain't Necessarily So: An Essay Review of *Intelligent Design Creationism and Its Critics: Philosophical, Theological, and Scientific Perspectives*." *Philosophy of Science* 71: 593–604.

Namba, Mitsuyoshi, Toshio Iwakura, Rimei Nishimura, Kohei Akazawa, Munehide Matsuhisa, Yoshihito Atsumi, Jo Satoh, and Toshimasa Yamauchi. 2018. "The Current Status of Treatment-Related Severe Hypoglycemia in Japanese Patients with Diabetes Mellitus: A Report from the Committee on a Survey of Severe Hypoglycemia in the Japan Diabetes Society." *Journal of Diabetes Investigation* 9 (3): 642–56.

Namihira, Emiko 波平 恵美子. 2005. 「からだの文化人類学—変貌する日本人の身体観」 [*Anthropology of the Body: The Changing Japanese View of the Body*.] Tokyo: Taishukan.

Nanri, Akiko, Tetsuya Mizue, Mitsuhiko Noda, Yoshihiko Takahashi, Masayuki Kato, Manami Inoue, Shoichiro Tsugane. 2010. "Rice Intake and Type 2 Diabetes in Japanese Men and Women: the Japan Public Health Center–Based Prospective Study." *American Journal of Clinical Nutrition* 92 (6): 1468–77.

Neville, Susan E., Kristina S. Boye, William S. Montgomery, Kazuya Iwamoto Masato Okamura, and Risa P. Hayes. 2009. "Diabetes in Japan: a Review of Disease Burden and Approaches to Treatment." *Diabetes/Metabolism Research and Reviews* 25 (8): 705–16.

Nigenda, Gustavo, Enrique Cifuentes, and Warren Hill. 2004. "Knowledge and Practice of Traditional Medicine in Mexico: A Survey of Healthcare Practitioners." *International Journal of Occupational and Environmental Health* 10 (4): 416–20.

Norbeck, Edward, and Margaret Lock, eds. 1987. *Health, Illness, and Medical Care in Japan: Cultural and Social Dimensions.* Honolulu: University of Hawaii Press.

Oberländer, Christian. 2005. "The Rise of Western 'Scientific Medicine' in Japan: Bacteriology and Beriberi." In *Building a Modern Japan: Science, Technology, and Medicine in the Meiji Era and Beyond*, edited by Morris Low, 13–36. New York: Palgrave Macmillan.

OECD Data. 2006. *OECD Health Data 2006: Statistics and Indicators.*

Office of Technology Assessment. 1978. "Assessing the Efficacy and Safety of Medical Technologies." *ota.fas.org.* Retrieved June 21, 2018 (http://ota.fas.org/reports/7805.pdf).

Ogasawara, Yuko. 1998. *Office Ladies and Salaried Men.* Berkeley: University of California Press.

Ohman-Strickland, P. A., A. John Orzano, Shawna V. Hudson, Leif I. Solberg, Barbara DiCiccio-Bloom, Dena O'Malley, Alfred F. Tallia, Bijal A. Balasubramanian, and Benjamin F. Crabtree. 2008. "Quality of Diabetes Care in Family Medicine Practices: Influence of Nurse-Practitioners and Physician's Assistants" *Annals of Family Medicine* 6: 14–22.

Ohnuki-Tierney, Emiko. 1984. *Illness and Culture in Contemporary Japan.* Cambridge: Cambridge University Press.

Oishi, Mariko, Katsuya Yamazaki, Fuminobu Okuguchi, Hidekatsu Sugimoto, Azuma Kanatsuka, and Atsunori Kashiwagi. 2014. "Changes in Oral Antidiabetic Prescriptions and Improved Glycemic Control During the Years 2002-2011 in Japan." *Journal of Diabetes Investigation* 5 (5): 581–87.

Ortloff, Debora Hinderliter, and Christopher J. Frey. 2007. "Blood Relatives: Language, Immigration, and Education of Ethnic Returnees in Germany and Japan." *Comparative Education Review.* 51 (4): 447–70.

Otsubo, Sumiko. 2005. "The Female Body and Eugenic Thought in Meiji Japan." In *Building a Modern Japan: Science, Technology, and Medicine in the Meiji Era and Beyond*, edited by Morris Low, 61–81. New York: Palgrave Macmillan.

Parthasarathy, Shobita. 2012. *Building Genetic Medicine: Breast Cancer, Technology, and the Comparative Politics of Health Care.* Cambridge, MA: MIT Press.

Payer, Lynn. 1988. *Medicine and Culture: Varieties of Treatment in the U.S., England, West Germany, and France.* New York: Henry Holt.

———. 1996. *Medicine and Culture.* New York: Henry Holt.

Pearlin, Leonard I., Elizabeth G. Menaghan, Morton A. Lieberman, and Joseph T. Mullan. 1981. "The Stress Process." *Journal of Health and Social Behavior* 22 (4): 337–56.

Peyrot, M., R. R. Rubin, T. Lauritzen, F. J. Snoek, D. R. Matthews, and S. E. Skovlund. 2005. "Psychosocial Problems and Barriers to Improved Diabetes Management: Results of the Cross-National Diabetes Attitudes, Wishes and Needs (DAWN) Study." *Diabetic Medicine: a Journal of the British Diabetic Association* 22 (10): 1379–85.

Pierce, Penny F., and Frank D. Hicks. 2001. "Patient Decision-Making Behavior: An Emerging Paradigm for Nursing Science." *Nursing Research* 50 (5): 267–274.

Pieterse, Jan Nederveen. 2004. *Globalization and Culture: Global Mélange.* Lanham, MD: Rowman & Littlefield.

Pollan, Michael. 2009. *In Defense of Food: An Eater's Manifesto*. New York: Penguin.

Poss, Jane, and Mary Ann Jezewski. 2002. "The Role and Meaning of *Susto* in Mexican-Americans' Explanatory Model of Type 2 Diabetes." *Medical Anthropology Quarterly* 16 (3): 360–77.

Reimann, Joachim O. F., Gregory A. Talavera, Michelle Salmon, Joseph A. Nuñez, and Roberto J. Velasquez. 2004. "Cultural Competence among Physicians Treating Mexican-Americans Who Have Diabetes: A Structural Model." *Social Science and Medicine* 59: 2195–2205.

Richardson, Theresa R. 1989. *The Century of the Child*. Albany: State University of New York Press, 1989.

Rickheim, Patti L., Todd W. Weaver, Jill L. Flader, and David M. Kendall. 2002. "Assessment of Group Versus Individual Diabetes Education." *Diabetes Care* 25 (2): 269–80.

Ritzer, George. 1993. *The McDonaldization of Society*. London: Sage.

Rizza, Robert, Robert A. Vigersky, Helena W. Rodbard, and Paul W. Ladenson. 2003. "A Model to Determine Workforce Needs for Endocrinologists in the United States Until 2020." *Diabetes Care* 26 (5): 1545–52.

Rock, Melanie. 2003. "Death, Taxes, Public Opinion, and the Midas Touch of Mary Tyler Moore: Accounting for Promises by Politicians to Help Avert and Control Diabetes." *Medical Anthropology Quarterly* 17 (2): 200–32.

———. 2005. "Diabetes Portrayals in North American Print Media: A Qualitative and Quantitative Analysis." *American Journal of Public Health* 95 (10): 1832–8.

Rose, Nikolas. 2007a. *The Politics of Life Itself*. Princeton: Princeton University Press.

———. 2007b. "Beyond Medicalisation." *Lancet* 369: 700–702.

Rosenstock, I. M. 1990. "The Health Belief Model: Explaining Health Behavior through Expectancies." In *Health Behavior and Health Education: Theory, Research, and Practice*, edited by K. Glantz, F. M. Lewis, and B. K. Rimer, 33–62. San Francisco: Jossey-Bass.

Roter Debra L., Moira Stewart, Samuel M. Putnam, Mack Lipkin, Jr., William Stiles, and Thomas S. Inui. 1997. "Communication Patterns of Primary Care Physicians." *Journal of the American Medical Association* 277 (4): 350–56.

Rubin, Alan. 2009. *Diabetes for Dummies*. Hoboken, NJ: John Wiley.

Saarmann, Lemby, JoAnn Daugherty, and Barbara Riegel. 2000. "Patient Teaching to Promote Behavioral Change." *Nursing Outlook* 48 (6): 281–87.

Sakai, Ryosuke, Y. Hashimoto, E. Ushigome, A. Miki, T. Okamura, M. Matsugasumi, T. Fukuda, et al. 2018. "Late-Night-Dinner Is Associated with Poor Glycemic Control in People with Type 2 Diabetes: The KAMOGAWA-DM Cohort Study." *Endocrine Journal* 65 (4): 395–402.

Sakane, Naoki, Juichi Sato, Kazuyo Tsushita, Satoru Tsujii, Kazuhiko Kotani, Kokoro Tsuzaki, Makoto Tominaga, et al. 2011. "Prevention of Type 2 Diabetes in a Primary Healthcare Setting: Three-Year Results of Lifestyle Intervention in Japanese Subjects with Impaired Glucose Tolerance." *BMC Public Health* 11 (1): 40.

Sakurai, Hideya. 2003. "Healthy Japan 21." *Journal of the Japan Medical Association* 46 (2): 47–49.

Santiago-Irizarry, Vilma. 2001. *Medicalizing Ethnicity: The Construction of Latino Identity in a Psychiatric Setting.* Ithaca, NY: Cornell University Press.

Sato, Junko, Akio Kanazawa, Chie Hatae, Sumiko Makita, Koji Komiya, Tomoaki Shimizu, Fuki Ikeda, et al. 2017a. "One Year Follow-Up After a Randomized Controlled Trial of a 130 G/Day Low-Carbohydrate Diet in Patients with Type 2 Diabetes Mellitus and Poor Glycemic Control." *PLOS ONE* 12 (12): e0188892.

Sato, Junko, Akio Kanazawa, Sumiko Makita, Chie Hatae, Koji Komiya, Tomoaki Shimizu, Fuki Ikeda, et al. 2017b. "A Randomized Controlled Trial of 130 G/Day Low-Carbohydrate Diet in Type 2 Diabetes with Poor Glycemic Control." *Clinical Nutrition* 36 (4): 992–1000.

Scheffler, Richard M., Stephen P. Hinshaw, Sepideh Modrek, and Peter Levine. 2007. "The Global Market for ADHD Medications." *Health Affairs* 26 (2): 450–57.

Schoenberg, Nancy, Elaine Drew, Eleanor Palo Stoller, and Cary Kart. 2005. "Situating Stress: Lessons from Lay Discourses on Diabetes." *Medical Anthropology Quarterly* 19 (2): 171–93.

Schouten, Barbara C., Ludwien Meeuwesen, Fred Tromp, and Hans A. M. Harmsen. 2007. "Cultural Diversity in Patient Participation: The Influence of Patients' Characteristics and Doctors' Communication Behavior." *Patient Education and Counseling* 67 (1–2): 214–23.

Schuerkens, Ulrike. 2003. "The Sociological and Anthropological Study of Globalization and Localization." *Current Sociology* 51: 209–22.

Seley, Jane Jeffrie, Phyllis Furst, Terry Gray, Donna Jornsay, and Nancy Reilly Wohl. 1999. "The Diabetes Nurse Practitioner: Promoting Partnerships in Care." *Diabetes Spectrum* 12 (2): 113–17.

Simpson, R. W., J. E. Shaw, and P. Z. Zimmet. 2003. "The Prevention of Type 2 Diabetes—Lifestyle Change or Pharmacotherapy? A Challenge for the 21st Century." *Diabetes Research and Clinical Practice* 59 (3): 165–80.

Shibaike, Nobuaki, Osamu Utsunomiya, Shin Ushiro, Tomoko Takamiya, and Akitsugu Ohuchi. 2002. "5. Action by Ministry of Health, Labor and Welfare National Health Promotion in the 21st Century 'Health Japan 21'." *Internal Medicine* 41 (1):70–71.

Solodky, Carrie, Hegang Chen, Paul K. Jones, William Katcher, and Duncan Neuhauser. 1998. "Patients as Partners in Clinical Research: A Proposal for Applying Quality Improvement Methods to Patient Care." *Medical Care* 36 (8): AS13–AS20.

Sone, H., and N. Yamada. 2010. "The Japan Diabetes Complications Study (JDCS)." [In Japanese.] *Nippon Rinsho* 68 (5): 865–71.

Sontag, Susan. 1978. *Illness as Metaphor.* London: Allen Lane.

Spann, Stephen J., Paul A. Nutting, and James M. Galliher, Kevin A. Peterson, Valory N. Pavlik, L. Miriam Dickinson, and Robert J. Volk. 2006. "Management of Type 2 Diabetes in the Primary Care Setting: A Practice-Based Research Network Study." *Annals of Family Medicine* 4 (10): 23–31.

Spencer, Karen L. 2018. "Transforming Patient Compliance Research in an Era of Biomedicalization." *Journal of Health and Social Behavior* 59 (2): 170–84.

Spero, David. 2006. *Diabetes: Sugar-Coated Crisis: Who Gets It, Who Profits, and How to Stop It.* Gabriola, BC: New Society Publishers.

Stake, Robert E. 2005. "Qualitative Case Studies." In *The Sage Handbook of Qualitative Research*, edited by Norman K. Denzin and Yvonna S. Lincoln, 443–66. Thousand Oaks, CA: Sage.

Starr, Paul. 1982. *The Social Transformation of American Medicine*. New York: Basic Books.

Strauss, Anselm. 1987. *Qualitative Analysis for Social Scientists*. Cambridge: Cambridge University Press.

Strauss, Anselm, and Juliet Corbin. 1990. *Basics of Qualitative Research: Grounded Theory Procedures and Techniques*. Newbury Park, CA: Sage.

Striegel-Moore, Ruth H., Debra L. Franko, Douglas Thompson, Sadra Affenito, Alexis May, and Helena C. Kraemer. 2008. "Exploring the Typology of Night Eating Syndrome." *International Journal of Eating Disorders* 41 (5): 411–18.

Sun, Qi, Donna Spiegelman, Rob M. van Dam, Michelle D. Holmes, Vasanti S. Malik, Walter C. Willett, and Frank B. Hu. 2010. "White Rice, Brown Rice, and Risk of Type 2 Diabetes in U.S. Men and Women." *Archives of Internal Medicine* 170: 961–9.

Sunday, Julie, John Eyles, and Ross Upshur. 2001. "Applying Aristotle's Doctrine of Causation to Aboriginal and Biomedical Understandings of Diabetes." *Culture, Medicine and Psychiatry* 25 (1): 63.

Swidler, Ann. 1986. "Culture in Action: Symbols and Strategies." *American Sociological Review* 51 (2): 273–86.

Tabuchi, Hiroko. 2009. "Why Japan's Cell Phones Haven't Gone Global." *New York Times*. July 19, B1.

Tamayo-Sarver, Joshua H., Susan W. Hinze, Rita K. Cydulka, and David W. Baker. 2003. "Racial and Ethnic Disparities in Emergency Department Analgesic Prescription." *American Journal of Public Health* 93 (12): 2067–73.

Tanaka, Nagaaki, Daisuke Yabe, Kenta Murotani, Shinji Ueno, Hitoshi Kuwata, Yoshiyuki Hamamoto, Takeshi Kurose, et al. 2018. "Mental Distress and Health-Related Quality of Life among Type 1 and Type 2 Diabetes Patients Using Self-Monitoring of Blood Glucose: A Cross-Sectional Questionnaire Study in Japan." *Journal of Diabetes Investigation*. Preprint before publication. DOI: 10.1111/jdi.12827.

Tierney, Lawrence M., Jr. 1994. "An Experience in Japanese Academic Medicine." *Western Journal of Medicine* 160 (2):139–45.

Timmermans, Stefan, and Rene Almeling. 2009. "Objectification, Standardization, and Commodification in Health Care: A Conceptual Readjustment." *Social Science and Medicine* 69 (1): 21–27.

Timmermans, Stefan, and Steven Epstein. 2010. "A World of Standards but Not a Standard World: Toward a Sociology of Standards and Standardization." *Annual Review of Sociology* 36 (1): 69–89.

Traphagan, John W. 2004. *The Practice of Concern: Ritual, Well-Being, and Aging in Rural Japan*. Chapel Hill, NC: Carolina Academic Press.

Traphagan, John W., and L. Keith Brown. 2002. "Fast Food and Intergenerational Commensality in Japan: New Styles and Old Patterns." *Ethnology* 41 (2): 119–34.

Triendl, Robert, and Davis Swinbanks. 1997. "Japan's Life Sciences Take Integrated Road." *Nature* 388: 216.

Tsuda, Takeyuki. 2003. *Strangers in the Ethnic Homeland: Japanese Brazilian Return Migration in Transnational Perspective.* New York: Columbia University Press.

Tsukimoto, You. 2008. 「日本人の脳に主語はいらない」 [*The Japanese Brain Doesn't Require a Grammatical Subject.*] Tokyo: Tankoubon.

Tsunoda, Tadanobu. 角田 忠信. 1978. 日本人の脳—脳の働きと東西の文化 大修館書店 [*The Japanese Brain.*] Tokyo: Taishuukanshoten.

Tsuruoka, Koki, Yuko Tsuruoka, Manabu Yoshimura, Koyu Imai, Satoko Sekiguchi, Junichi Mise, Yasuhiro Asai, Naoki Nago, and Masahiro Igarashi. 1996. "Evidence Based General Practice. Drug Treatment in General Practice in Japan Is Evidence Based." *British Medical Journal* 313 (7049): 114–15.

Tu, Ha T., and Ann S. O'Malley. 2007. "Exodus of Male Physicians from Primary Care Drives Shift to Specialty Practice." Tracking Report 17. Center for Studying Health System Change.

Udagawa, Koko, Miki Miyoshi, and Nobuo Yoshiike. 2008. "Mid-Term Evaluation of 'Health Japan 21'." *Asia Pacific Journal of Clinical Nutrition* 17 (S2): 445–52.

Vaughn, Nicole Angela. 2004. "Impact of Insurance Status on Health Care Utilization and Quality of Self-Care among Ethnic Minorities with Type 2 Diabetes." Ph.D. dissertation. Uniformed Services University of the Health Sciences—Maryland.

Waitzkin, Howard. 1989. "A Critical Theory of Medical Discourse: Ideology, Social Control, and the Processing of Social Context in Medical Encounters." *Journal of Health and Social Behavior* 30 (2): 220–39.

Walsh, Michele, Murray Katz, and Lee Sechrest. 2002. "Unpacking Cultural Factors in Adaptation to Type 2 Diabetes Mellitus." *Medical Care* 40 (1): 129–39.

Watanabe, Shoichi. 1954. 「日本語の心」 [*The Heart of the Japanese Language.*] 厳冬者。

Whittemore, R., S. K. Chase, C. L. Mandle, and C. Roy. 2002. "Lifestyle Change in Type 2 Diabetes: A Process Model." *Nursing Research* 51 (1): 18–25.

Whyte, Susan Reynolds, Sjaak Van Der Geest, and Anita Hardon. 2002. *The Social Lives of Medicines.* Cambridge: Cambridge University Press.

Williams, Simon J., Clive Seale, Sharon Boden, Pam Lowe, and Deborah Lynn Steinberg. 2009. "Waking Up to Sleepiness." In *Pharmaceuticals and Society: Critical Discourses and Debates*, edited by Simon J. Williams, Jonathan Gabe, and Peter Davis, 25–40. Chichester: Wiley-Blackwell.

Williams Simon J., Paul Martin, and Jonathan Gabe. 2011. "The Pharmaceuticalisation of Society? A Framework for Analysis." *Sociology of Health and Illness* 33 (5): 710–725.

Woodall, Brian. 1997. "Japan's Double Standards: Technical Standards and U.S.–Japan Economic Relations." In *Japan's Technical Standards: Implications for Global Trade and Competitiveness*, edited by John R. McIntyre, 145–61. Westport, CT: Quorum Books.

Yamada, Satoru. 2017. "Paradigm Shifts in Nutrition Therapy for Type 2 Diabetes." *Keio Journal of Medicine* 66 (3): 33–43.

Yamamoto, Takuya, Shota Moyama, and Hideki Yano. 2017. "Effect of a Newly-Devised Nutritional Guide Based on Self-Efficacy for Patients with Type 2

Diabetes in Japan over 2 Years: 1-Year Intervention and 1-Year Follow-Up Studies." *Journal of Diabetes Investigation* 8 (2): 195–200.

Yamaoka, Kazue, and Toshiro Tango. 2005. "Efficacy of Lifestyle Education to Prevent Type 2 Diabetes: A Meta-Analysis of Randomized Controlled Trials." *Diabetes Care* 28 (11): 2780–6.

Yoro, Rika 養老 孟司. 1996. 「日本人の身体観の歴史」[*History of the Japanese View of the Body*]. Tokyo: Hozokan.

Yoshino, Kosaku. 2005. *Cultural Nationalism in Contemporary Japan: A Sociological Enquiry*. London: Routledge.

Yoshioka, Eiji 吉岡 英治. 2010. 「SW2010オープニング行事 北海道大学「持続可能な発 展」国際シンポジウム：ひとり一人がすこやかに人間ら しく生きる社会を目指して：わたしたちが直面する危機 の原因を包括的に探る」分科会4：高齢社会の健康と介護：幸せとは?. 平成22年10月26日(火). 北海道大学学術交 流会館, 札幌市.

Yoshioka, Narihito, Hitoshi Ishii, Naoko Tajima, Yasuhiko Iwamoto, and the DAWN Japan Group. 2014. "Differences in Physician and Patient Perceptions About Insulin Therapy for Management of Type 2 Diabetes: the DAWN Japan Study." *Current Medical Research and Opinion* 30 (2): 177–83.

Yudkin, John, Kasia Lipska, and Victor Montori. 2011. "The Idolatry of the Surrogate." *British Medical Journal* 343: d7995.

Zola, I. K. 1972. "Medicine as an Institution of Social Control." *Sociological Review* 20: 487–504.

Index

Organisation for Economic Co-operation and Development (OECD), 4–5

"paleofantasy," 36, 37
Parthasarathy, Shobita, 51
paternalistic treatment: in Japan, 93–97, 100–101, 103; in United States, 75, 77–79, 82, 84–86
patient-centered treatment: in Japan, 95–97, 100–102, 108; in United States, 75, 77–80 passim, 82, 85, 86, 90, 97, 100
prediabetes states, 3, 26–27, 121–22
pharmaceuticals, 5, 15, 20, 22, 89, 90, 131; pharmaceuticalization, 23–24
pharmacotherapy, 27
pre-illness concerns and programs, 25–28
psychiatry, 22

rice, 1, 4, 6, 65, 66, 68–69
Rock, Melanie, 38, 46, 49, 142n1
Rose, Nikolas, 31, 130
Rubin, Alan, 39

self-management, 13, 76, 83, 92, 94, 104–7 passim, 131
Sontag, Susan, 46
speech registers, 98, 100–101
Starr, Paul, 7–8
Sugita, 16
Swidler, Ann, 32, 34

Takeshi, Beat, 28–29
technoscientization of health practice, 29–30, 31–32

Tierney, Lawrence M., 18
traditional and alternative medicine, 9, 21, 42, 102; *kampo*, 21, 72
triglycerides, 29
type 1 diabetes, 41, 42–45, 142n4
type 2 diabetes: causes and risk factors of, 2, 3, 6, 38–39; delayed diagnosis of, 3, 107–8, 120; depression and, 81–82; incurable nature of, 106–7, 213; Internet and, 100, 102–3; popular books on, 38–39, 142n2; pre-illness focus on, 26; as spiritual indictment, 11; treatments for, 4–7, 14. *See also* food and diabetes; Japan and type 2 diabetes; obesity; United States and type 2 diabetes

United States: health care system in, 5, 9–11, 141n2; health data collection in, 27; health visits frequency in, 4–5; medical profession in, 20, 75–91; public health interventions in, 3–4; risk and responsibility in, 32, 34, 46–47, 83, 132; tropes of identity in, 35; the uninsured in, 11
United States and type 2 diabetes: origin stories of, 12–13, 28, 34, 36–50; pessimistic expectations and, 87–91, 102, 109; pre-illness focus and, 27; provider-patient relationship and, 4–7, 75–91; rates for, 2, 64

White, Kerr, 18–19

Yamanaka, Shinya, 10

Zuk, Marlene, 36

Studies in Social Medicine

NANCY M. P. KING, GAIL E. HENDERSON, AND JANE STEIN, eds., *Beyond Regulations: Ethics in Human Subjects Research* (1999).

LAURIE ZOLOTH, *Health Care and the Ethics of Encounter: A Jewish Discussion of Social Justice* (1999).

SUSAN M. REVERBY, ed., *Tuskegee's Truths: Rethinking the Tuskegee Syphilis Study* (2000).

BEATRIX HOFFMAN, *The Wages of Sickness: The Politics of Health Insurance in Progressive America* (2000).

MARGARETE SANDELOWSKI, *Devices and Desires: Gender, Technology, and American Nursing* (2000).

KEITH WAILOO, *Dying in the City of the Blues: Sickle Cell Anemia and the Politics of Race and Health* (2001).

JUDITH ANDRE, *Bioethics as Practice* (2002).

CHRIS FEUDTNER, *Bittersweet: Diabetes, Insulin, and the Transformation of Illness* (2003).

ANN FOLWELL STANFORD, *Bodies in a Broken World: Women Novelists of Color and the Politics of Medicine* (2003).

LAWRENCE O. GOSTIN, *The AIDS Pandemic: Complacency, Injustice, and Unfulfilled Expectations* (2004).

ARTHUR A. DAEMMRICH, *Pharmacopolitics: Drug Regulation in the United States and Germany* (2004).

CARL ELLIOTT AND TOD CHAMBERS, eds., *Prozac as a Way of Life* (2004).

STEVEN M. STOWE, *Doctoring the South: Southern Physicians and Everyday Medicine in the Mid-Nineteenth Century* (2004).

ARLEEN MARCIA TUCHMAN, *Science Has No Sex: The Life of Marie Zakrzewska, M.D.* (2006).

MICHAEL H. COHEN, *Healing at the Borderland of Medicine and Religion* (2006).

KEITH WAILOO, JULIE LIVINGSTON, AND PETER GUARNACCIA, eds., *A Death Retold: Jesica Santillan, the Bungled Transplant, and Paradoxes of Medical Citizenship* (2006).

MICHELLE T. MORAN, *Colonizing Leprosy: Imperialism and the Politics of Public Health in the United States* (2007).

KAREY HARWOOD, *The Infertility Treadmill: Feminist Ethics, Personal Choice, and the Use of Reproductive Technologies* (2007).

CARLA BITTEL, *Mary Putnam Jacobi and the Politics of Medicine in Nineteenth-Century America* (2009).

SAMUEL KELTON ROBERTS JR., *Infectious Fear: Politics, Disease, and the Health Effects of Segregation* (2009).

LOIS SHEPHERD, *If That Ever Happens to Me: Making Life and Death Decisions after Terri Schiavo* (2009).

MICAL RAZ, *What's Wrong with the Poor? Psychiatry, Race, and the War on Poverty* (2013).

JOHANNA SCHOEN, *Abortion after* Roe (2015).

NANCY TOMES, *Remaking the American Patient: How Madison Avenue and Modern Medicine Turned Patients into Consumers* (2016).

MARA BUCHBINDER, MICHELE RIVKIN-FISH, AND REBECCA L. WALKER, eds., *Understanding Health Inequalities and Justice: New Conversations across the Disciplines* (2016).

MURIEL R. GILLICK, *Old and Sick in America: The Journey through the Health Care System* (2017).

MICHAEL E. STAUB, *The Mismeasure of Minds: Debating Race and Intelligence between* Brown *and "The Bell Curve"* (2018).

MARI ARMSTRONG-HOUGH, *Biomedicalization and the Practice of Culture: Globalization and Type 2 Diabetes in the United States and Japan* (2018).

www.ingramcontent.com/pod-product-compliance
Lightning Source LLC
Chambersburg PA
CBHW030333270326
41926CB00010B/1610